How to Walk in Stilettos

Original title:

Comment Marcher sur des Stilettos

Manuel de survie pour les accros aux chaussures

Join Sixtine Garnier on Instagram :
@sixtinegarnier

Sixtine Garnier

How to Walk in Stilettos

A Survival Guide for Shoe Addicts

Translated from French by Sarita Jannin

CreateSpace Independent Publishing Platform, USA

ISBN: 978-1974395910

For all shoe addicts…
And for the designers who make us dream…

- Contents -

- Disclaimer -

The information in this book is for informative purposes only and should in no case be considered medical or pharmaceutical advice. This information and its use therefore in no way incur the liability of the author, the illustrator, or the publisher. In continuing to read this book, you agree to the present liability disclaimer for the author, the illustrator and the publisher, without exonerating yourself or claiming to benefit from a derogation of any nature whatsoever. By using the information contained in this book, you are solely responsible for the consequences of your actions.

The cosmetic formulas and the sequence of stretches and exercises chosen are original works protected by copyright and intellectual property law, which cannot be used for commercial purposes without the prior and restrictive consent of the author and the publisher. Any total or partial reproduction, distribution, or modification of this work by any process whatsoever, known or planned, is strictly prohibited without the prior written consent of the author and illustrator.

- Introduction -

Deciding to spend the day walking about in high heels is no small matter... Well, okay, that's not quite true. It is a quick decision to make, and sometimes we even choose the pair of stilettos we want to wear for the day before deciding on the outfit that sets them off best.

But after spending several hours perched on our beloved pair of heels, our body is often aching and our feet are bruised. In this handbook, which has been especially designed for all those shoe addicts out there, you will find all sorts of tips and tricks to relieve the pain, recognize the different types of heels, learn how to walk about gracefully on your favorite pair of pumps, and prepare your own miracle formulas… but that's not all!

The last part of this book teaches you how to strengthen, tone, and stretch out all the parts of your body that are used when wearing heels.

All about Shoes

"Men often tell me that I have saved their marriage. They've spent a fortune on my shoes, but it's always cheaper than a divorce."

Manolo Blahnik

- Chapter 1 -
The History of Shoes

"Show me your shoes, and I will tell you who you are." A pair of shoes can tell you a lot about the wearer. Her tastes, her culture, her socio-economic status, whether she takes care of her belongings, her sense of detail... But do you know how shoes, these simple pieces of assembled leather and fabric, first developed? And why they have gained such a growing place in our wardrobes and society? Did you know they reflect the evolution of our values and culture?

When people first began wearing shoes, it wasn't for aesthetic reasons, but for purely practical reasons—to protect themselves from contact with the ground to avoid injuries and the cold. The first shoes were made from bark or wood to protect the soles of the feet. Let's go on a quick tour together of the history of shoes throughout the ages...

Around 4,000 BC:

The inhabitants of the colder climates tied furs around their feet, ankles, and calves.

In hot climates, people protected themselves from the

burning soil by tying palm leaves to the soles of their feet.

In the Alps, the remains of a pair of leather shoes have been found, which probably belonged to a Neolithic hunter.

Antiquity:

Sandals were THE fashion in Greece, Egypt, and the Roman Empire.

To begin with, in ancient Egypt, sandals were only worn by gods and important figures (pharaohs, queens, high dignitaries, and priests). Until sandals reached the masses, people went about barefoot. The first platform shoes appeared and were reserved for... butchers so that their feet weren't soaked in blood.

In ancient Greece, sandals were only for high dignitaries. Women and the elderly wore closed, soft leather shoes, inspired by Persian tradition. Decoration and jewels on sandals was also regulated.

Under the Roman Empire, certain conventions had to be respected: the types of shoes to be worn according to social status, the way the shoes were decorated, ornaments, colors, and the number of straps holding the shoe in place (the higher the status, the greater the number of straps).

The Middle Ages:

Trade and exchange were developing and fashions began to change with new imports. The upper classes demonstrated their wealth by buying imported products, and carefully choosing the colors, styles, and fabrics of their clothes and shoes.

Shoes became closed and were made of skins or furs. Pointed shoes became fashionable. Regardless of foot measurements, the length of the tip of the shoe, known as the poulaine, indicated the social status and wealth of the wearer. Royalty would wear shoes up to about 20 inches long. The tips of the shoes were stiffened by padding them with hemp or moss.

Some people refused to wear shoes in sign of repentance and humility (the Saints were approached barefoot).

16th century:

It was winds of change across Europe at a societal, political, and intellectual level, and this was reflected in the changing fashions. In contrast with the Middle Ages, the tips of shoes now became wide and square.

But the height of the soles changed too. Nobody quite knows when platform shoes began to appear, but during the Renaissance, chopines became fashionable in Florence and

Venice, Italy. These platform shoes, measuring up to 24 inches in height, were inspired by oriental models. The main purpose of these shoes was to keep the bottom of the courtesans' dresses clean. Of course, the search for aesthetics is never far behind... The raised soles were made of light wood and covered with fabric, leather, and sometimes decorations. A lady would need good balance and the arm of a servant (or gallant escort) to wear these extravagant shoes.

Women began to adopt a new posture that made their hips sway, and their movements became more erotic.

Little by little, the front part of the chopines became lower and the shoes were easier to wear, the shape more similar to that of modern day shoes.

Catherine de' Medici was the first woman to import chopines from Italy to the French Court for her marriage with the Duke of Orléans, while Queen Mary I introduced them in England.

17th and early 18th century:

High-heeled shoes spread throughout the European nobility. The aristocrats of Louis XIV of France's court were considered closer to God and his representative, the King, and were therefore above the common people (both symbolically and physically by wearing heels).

These shoes, which were very unpractical to wear, and which didn't distinguish between the left foot and right foot, couldn't be worn by the common people who needed to be able to move about easily for work.

The heels were so high that women needed walking canes to help them move about. Skirts became shorter to reveal the ladies graceful feet and ankles, features that were accentuated by the high heels.

The richer a person and the higher their rank, the more sumptuous the decoration on their shoes with buckles, laces, ribbons, pearls, and precious stones. Only nobility was allowed to wear red heels.

The Baroque period influenced the fashion further: the originality and richness of the materials (velvet and silk), ornaments and embroidery, buckles and carefully crafted clips...

Late 18th - Early 19th century:

Wearing beautifully crafted shoes with buckles or high heels, were signs of aristocracy and were frowned upon during the French Revolution. Shoes became more sober and no longer had heels. All men were now considered equal, so everyone had to be at ground level. Ankle boots became fashionable.

It wasn't until the French Empire gained power that decorations, bows and ruffles were used to decorate shoes and boots again.

Late 19th century:

Beautiful shoes with calfskin uppers were the sign of the members of the ruling class, who did not perform manual work.

Meanwhile, women wore ankle boots with buttons or laces. For women only, mid-high heels reappeared among the French bourgeoisie. Heels were considered disreputable by some, symbols of sexuality, worn by the dancers of the French Cancan who were likened to prostitutes.

Early 20th century:

Fashions and styles multiplied throughout the century, as did the use of new materials, thanks to the development of new techniques and industry. Shoes were becoming more democratic.

1920s–1930s: society was evolving and fashion was too. Women were becoming more powerful and starting to want freedom, while still retaining their female identity. The lengths of skirts became shorter, ankle boots gave way to pumps, and heels became higher to flatter and sculpt the calves. Leather, in different colors, could now be coated in gold or silver.

***1930s to 1945*:** women wore wedge heels and platform shoes.

1950s: inspired by Christian Dior's New Look, pumps became more glamorous to set off bell skirts—heels became slimmer, and the spike heel was born. To make the wooden heels stronger, and lighter than steel heels, metal rods were inserted into them. At first, only "disreputable" women (or Hollywood vamps) wore spike heels, which were considered the ultimate sex symbol.

In the teenage girls' fashion popularized by Audrey Hepburn, pumps were abandoned in favor of ballet flats, which were worn with ankle grazer pants.

1960s: heels became lower and wider once again, both in the form of the vinyl boots worn with mini-skirts by Beatles fans, and the colorful sandals worn by hippies.

1970s: the grand return of colorful platform shoes and wedge heels with wide tips.

1980s: a combination of the fashions of the previous decades (pumps with buckles, wedge shoes, etc.) but at the same time a return to comfort, with the fashion for wearing sneakers in the city.

- Chapter 2 -
Six Designers who Revolutionized Shoes

Many have made a difference and many have been forgotten. It was difficult to decide which ones should feature in this mini-list. So I kept only six names: André Perugia for his avant-gardism, Roger Vivier for his heels, Rose Repetto for her mythical ballet shoes, Manolo Blahnik for his constantly evolving modernity, Giuseppe Zanotti for his "foot jewelry", and Christian Louboutin for his iconic soles. Of course, your six flagship names may be different. Each to their own. But I'll present you mine.

André Pérugia

The son of a shoemaker, André Perugia was born in Nice, France, in 1893 and decided to follow in his father's footsteps when he was only sixteen.

In 1921, after working with Paul Poiret (the great Art Deco fashion designer), André Pérugia opened his first boutique in Paris. From then one he began constantly seeking to renew genre and form. Some of his designs are tributes to the artists he most loved.

In 1933, he launched his Padova brand, which was uniquely distributed by the Saks Fifth Avenue stores, after the Americans hailed his innovative designs. His constant search for modernity continued until he retired in 1970. He died 7 years later.

"A woman's feet are a secret insight into her personality."
(André Perugia in his book *From Eve to Rita Hayworth)*

Some of André Pérugia's most famous models: the cubist sandal, the heel-less shoe, the spiral-heeled shoe, the sandal in tribute to Picasso, and the fish pump in tribute to Georges Braque.

Roger Vivier

Roger Vivier was born in 1903 and took studies in fine arts, specializing in sculpture, before turning to the world of shoes.

In 1930, Roger Vivier began designing custom made shoes for the great names of his time (Joséphine Baker, Mistinguett…). This led him to open his first boutique in Paris in 1937 and to set up his fashion house there in 1963.

Like André Pérugia, Roger Vivier was a precursor of his time: he used plastic (1945), created the ball heel (for Marlene Dietrich in 1953), invented the spike heel (1954), then the shock heel (1959), and finally the Virgule "comma" heel (1963), and he designed shoes for Catherine Deneuve in the film *Belle de Jour* (1965).

But he was also a symbol of French savoir-faire: in 1953, he was asked to design the shoes worn by Her Majesty Queen Elizabeth II at her coronation.

Rogier Vivier died on 2 October 1998 in Toulouse, France.

> *"Curves and lines have always fascinated me. I'll redo a design five hundred times to make sure the concept is accurate and respects the architecture of the foot."* (Roger Vivier)

Some of his emblematic designs: the spike heel, the shock heel, the Virgule or "comma" heel, the shoes designed for Queen Elizabeth II, and his Belle pumps.

Rose Repetto

Rose Repetto was born in 1907. Of Italian origin, she was the mother of Claude and Roland Petit. It was for Roland Petit, the famous dancer and choreographer, who trained at the Paris Opera, that she sewed her first pair of ballet shoes, which allowed great ease of movement and reduced injury due to their unrivalled comfort. Rose Repetto used a technique that the Repetto brand still uses today to manufacture its ballerina slippers and ballet shoes: the stitch and return technique.

Before long, Parisian dancers were all coming to her to buy both their ballet shoes and dance outfits. Her boutique, which opened in 1959, was frequented by Rudolf Nureyev, Maurice Béjart, and Mikhail Baryshnikov among many others.

In 1956, Brigitte Bardot asked Repetto to design ballerina shoes for her: the Cendrillon model was born, immortalized on Bridget Bardon in *And God Created Woman*. Rose Repetto then designed the Zizi model for her daughter-in-law, Zizi Jeanmaire, (a ballerina and lead revue artist). The singer, Serge Gainsbourg, also liked them so much that he became one of the symbols of the brand, as did Mick Jagger.

"Repetto forever!" (Serge Gainsbourg)

Rose Repetto died in 1984, and the brand was quiet for a while. Then from 1999, Repetto had a new upswing: ballerina shoes became popular again throughout the world, with new materials and cult styles.

Repetto, a brand combining tradition and novelty: Cendrillon ballerina shoes, the Zizi Oxford shoe, the Baya t-strap, and the Daren loafer.

Manolo Blahnik

Manolo Blahnik was born in the Canary Islands in 1942. He came to love fashion and shoes from an early age thanks to his mother who subscribed to several different magazines and made her own shoes.

Blahnik did studies to become an architect and then a theatrical scene painter (at the Ecole des Beaux-Arts and the Ecole du Louvre in France). Then, in the early 1970s, he became a photographer, but he still enjoyed sketching. He presented his many drawings to the chief editor of *Vogue* magazine, Diana Vreeland, who encouraged him to begin designing shoes. Soon after, Blahnik opened his first boutique. He was rapidly successful: sales grew and his boutiques multiplied. His name has been mentioned in various TV series (*Absolutely fabulous, Sex and the City...*) and in songs, and his designs have been worn in films (Sofia Coppola's *Marie-Antoinette* and *Twilight*).

From his studies in architecture, he learned attention to detail: his shoes needed to follow the curves of a woman's foot, without her suffering. There was no point in his designs being beautiful if they weren't comfortable.

> *"I like [shoes] that are exaggerated, and I like [shoes] that are eccentric, but you have to be comfortable. Otherwise, it's absurd. There's nothing charming about a woman who can't walk in her own shoes."*
>
> (Manolo Blahnik)

Real favorites: Ossie sandals, Campari Mary Janes, Climatida sandals, Hangisi pumps, Swan pumps, and Contun sandals.

Giuseppe Zanotti

Born in Italy in 1958 in one of the cradles of shoe manufacturing, Giuseppe Zanotti worked as a DJ by night and began rubbing shoulders in the world of shoes by becoming an independent designer for shoemaking workshops, and then a consultant for major fashion houses. In 1990, he began designing shoes for famous brands such as Dior and Cavalli.

In 1994, Zanotti presented his own line in New York: Giuseppe Zanotti Design was born. His success was immediate. The brand grew and was distributed in large luxury chain stores, before opening its own stores. Giuseppe Zanotti even bought the Vincini workshops, a brand he had worked for as a consultant a few years earlier.

Giuseppe Zanotti is considered the biggest name in "jewelry shoes." Chains, pearls, crystals, gem stones, and pieces of metal are often inserted in GZD footwear, the true signature of the brand.

Since the 2000s, Giuseppe Zanotti Design has been working with some of the biggest names in fashion to create ephemeral collections: Balmain, Vionnet, and Vera Wang. The brand has also been diversifying its range of designs with men's collections, leather goods (belts and handbags), tailor-made designs, ready-to-wear clothing, and jewelry.

"You can't design shoes if you only think of fashion. When I design, I dream" (Giuseppe Zanotti)

A few of the "jewels" of Giuseppe Zanotti Design: Rose, Coline, Belle, Choker, and Cruel Summer sandals...

Christian Louboutin

Born in Paris, France, on January 27, 1964, Christian Louboutin began designing shoes from his childhood, inspired by an image that remained engraved in his memory: that of a pair of pumps on a poster prohibiting spike heels that could scratch the wooden flooring at the Museum of African and Oceanic Arts.

He began selling some of his designs to the dancers at Folies Bergères, and then at other places such as the Palace. He then got an internship with Charles Jourdan, who was known for his spike heels, before designing some models for large fashion houses, and going on to create his own brand and open his first boutique in 1991.

Soon recognized for his designs, particularly by Anna Wintour, he set up another store in New York in 1993, and became a shoemaker for major fashion shows from 1995, as celebrities began snapping up his creations. In the 2000s, Christian Louboutin continued to develop his brand with a collection of bags and makeup.

Known for his famous red leather soles (the idea came to him when he painted the soles of one of his designs with his assistant's red Chanel nail varnish) and his famous range of pumps with dizzying heels, he is almost systematically quoted by women when asked: "Can you tell us the name of a famous shoe designer?"

"If you want to feel like a woman, wear heels. If you want to feel like a goddess, wear 4 inch heels." (Christian Louboutin)

A range of stilettos from Christian Louboutin, including among other models: Ron, Lady Peep, Fifi, Kid, Simple Pump, and Pigalle…

- Chapter 3 -
The Different Parts of the Heel and Sole

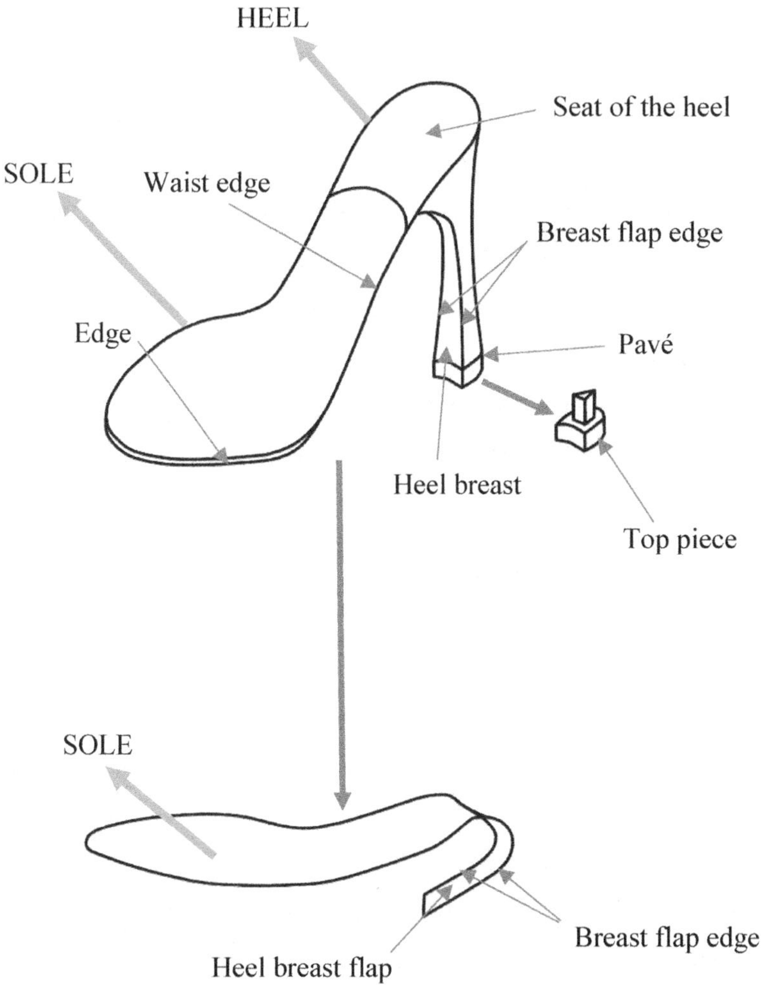

Legend:

- **Edge**: the outer surface of the sole.
- **Waist edge**: the part of the edge located at the arch of the foot.
- **Heel breast flap**: the back part of the sole that lies against the heel breast
- **Heel breast**: the forward facing part of the heel (which can be straight or concave).
- **Breast flap edge**: the parts that carry over from the heel breast flap (for a Louis heel) and the heel breast.
- **Seat of the heel**: the concave upper part of the heel.
- **Pavé:** the part of the heel that faces the ground and comes into contact with the top piece.
- **Top piece**: the durable layer under the heel that helps to absorb shocks and protect the bottom of the heel.

- Chapter 4 -
The Main Types of Heel and Sole

So you love shoes, but do you know the names of the different kinds of heels? Heels are defined by various criteria: height, shape (curvature and profile), and type of manufacture (coated, spool, etc.).

For example: a 3 inch spool heel

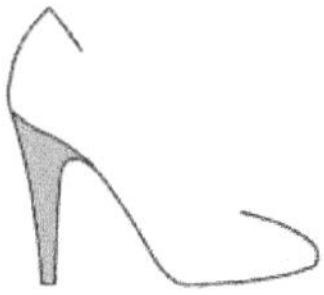

Spike heel: the heel tapers downward so the surface of the top piece is smaller than the rest of the heel.

Stiletto heel: a close cousin of spike heels, pin heels are thin throughout the length of the heel as far as the seat of the heel.

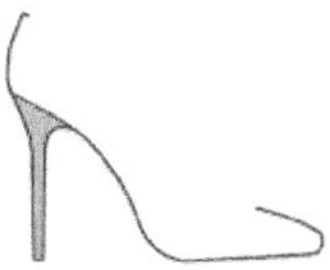

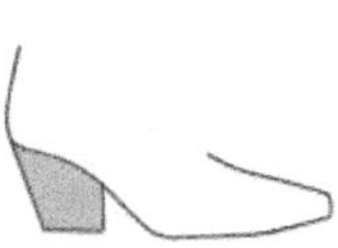

Cuban heel: the sides are straight but the back edge slopes forward.

Flared heel: the heel is wider at the bottom than at the top.

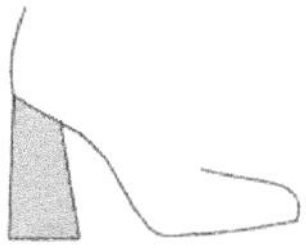

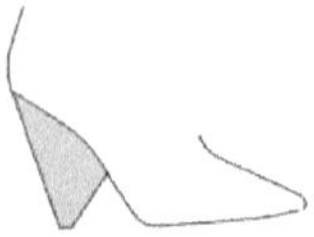

Cone heel: a triangular shaped profile, with the base situated under the seat of the heel.

Claw heel: the heel can vary in thickness, but is concave in a forward direction (from a side view).

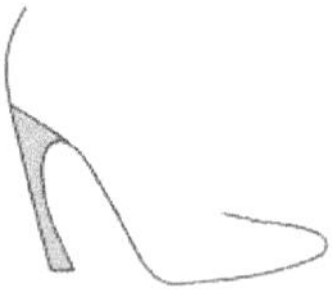

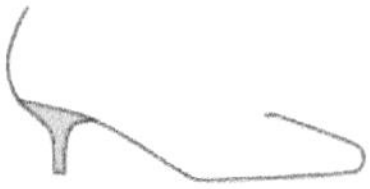

Kitten Heel: 1-2 inches in height, and relatively slim.

Block heel: the sides are straight and parallel.

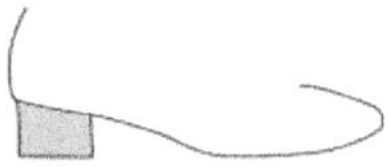

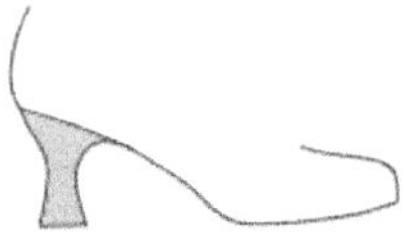

Spool heel: the heel is slimmer in the middle, giving it a flared appearance at the top piece.

Louis heels: a concave side profile, the heel breast is covered with an extension of the sole (known as the heel breast flap).

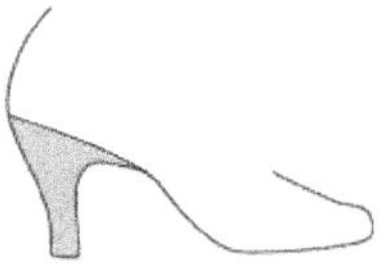

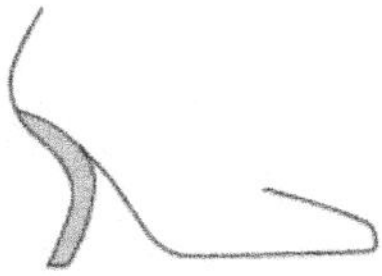

Comma heels: designed by Roger Vivier in 1963, these heels are convex in a forward direction.

Flat heel: there is a continuity between the sole and the heel.

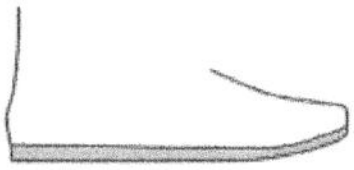

Low heel: there is only a thin layer of material (leather, for example) under the seat of the heel. It is THE heel for ballerina shoes.

French heel: the heel can be flat or high, with a concave heel breast.

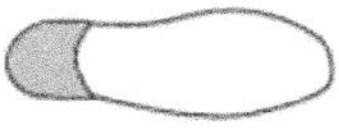

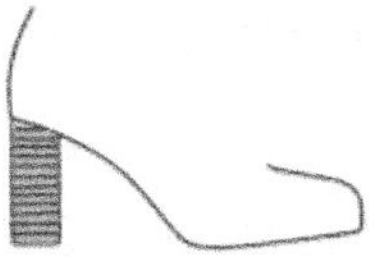

Stacked heel: this heel looks like it is made of several stacked layers (leather or imitation).

Coated heel: the heel is covered in an "envelope" of leather or fabric.

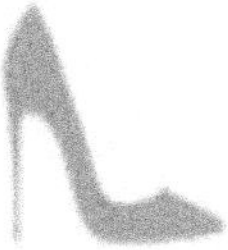

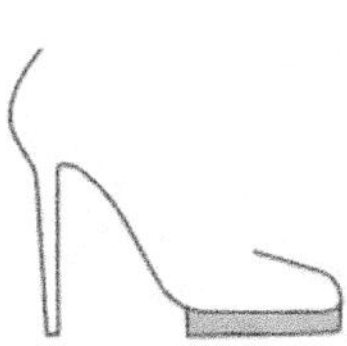

Platform heels: the height of the sole means that the front of the foot is raised above the ground. It can be combined with a wedge heel or a stiletto heel…

Scoop-wedge heel: almost identical to a wedge heel, but there is a discontinuity under the arch of the foot, before it reaches the base of the sole.

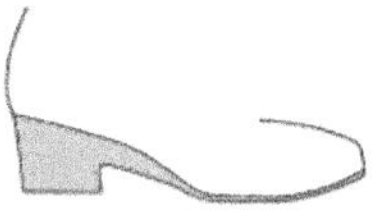

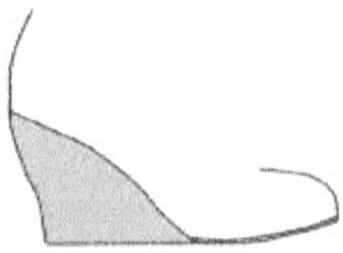

Wedge heel: from the side view, the heel continues smoothly under the arch of the foot until it reaches the base of the sole.

How is heel height defined?

Generally speaking, we talk about:

- flat heels when they are less than ½ an inch in height,
- low heels when they are around 1 inch in height,
- mid heels when they are around 2 inches in height,
- and high heels when they are over 3 inches in height (very high heels if they are taller than 3.5 inches).

- Chapter 5 -
The Different Styles of Shoe

Do you know the difference between your two pairs of black pumps? What is the name of that cut at the front of the foot? Now you know the different shapes of heels and soles, the following little guide is just what you need. (Of course, this little list is not exhaustive...)

Mary Janes

A strap across the instep, a heel of varying height, and a round or pointed tip. In France, these shoes are divided into two categories: “Mary Janes” for the more feminine, high-heeled styles, and “Babies” for the lower heeled, more child-like styles.

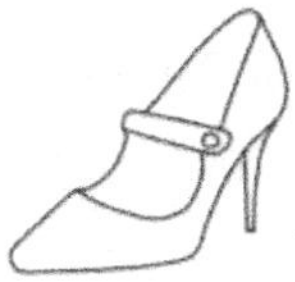

Mules

Only the front of the foot is covered. They can be closed or open toed.

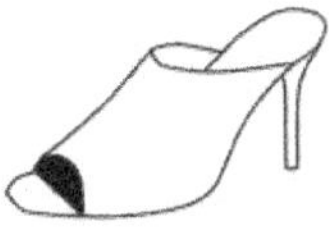

T-strap pumps

There is a transverse strap, with a perpendicular strap attached onto it that comes up to the middle of the instep.

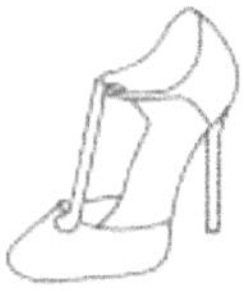

D'Orsays

Only the toes and heels are covered (and sometimes one of the two sides). They can be closed or open toed.

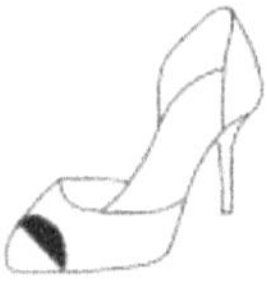

Jewel embellished pumps

These are covered (partially or entirely) in pearls or gem stones, often imitation.

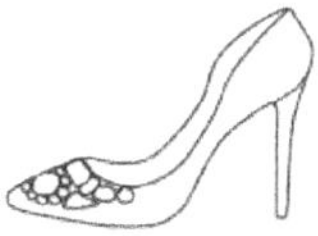

Cage Pumps

Multiple straps hold the foot in place.

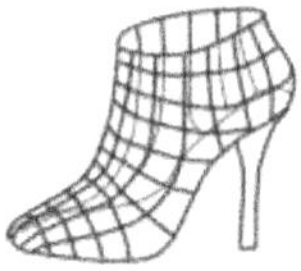

Crisscross pumps

The straps cross over on the instep.

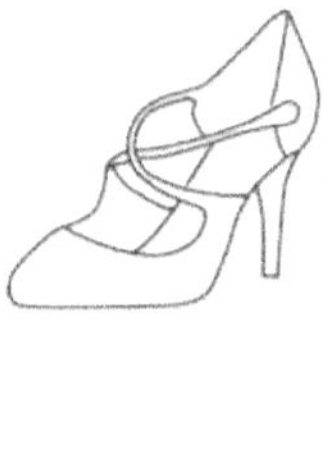

Slingbacks

A strap around the back of the foot holds it in place in the shoe.

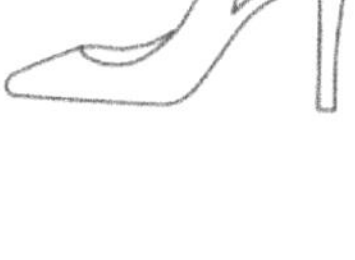

Gladiator sandals

These sandals are inspired by the shoes worn in Ancient Greece.

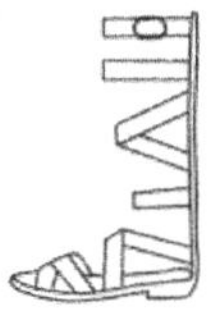

Tropeziennes

These sandals are easily recognizable for the distinctive arrangement of the straps.

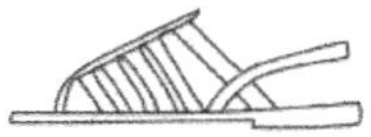

Thongs

There is a V-shaped strap between the first two toes. There is no other strap.

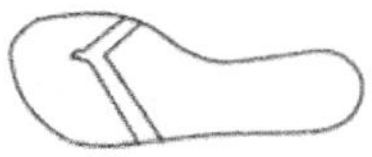

T-strap sandals

There is a strap between the toes which meets a transverse strap.

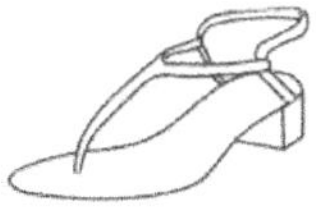

Espadrilles

Recognizable for their rope sole (hessian or hemp).

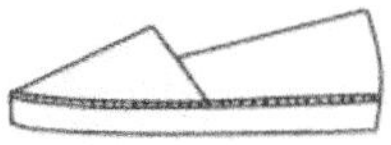

Ballerina shoes

Inspired by dance slippers, ballerina shoes have a very thin sole, with a flat or low heel.

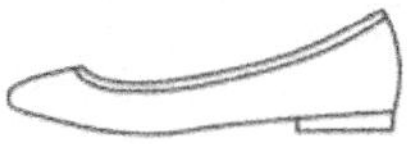

Slip-ons

Their main characteristic is that they are easy to slip on, for example with an elasticated opening.

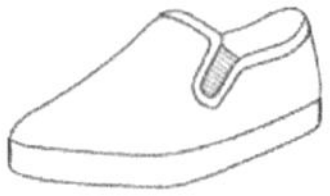

Slippers

A near cousin of moccasins, these shoes closely resemble indoor slippers, but can be worn outside.

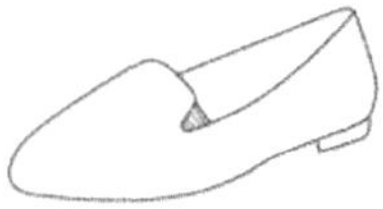

Moccasins/Loafers

A low, supple leather shoe.

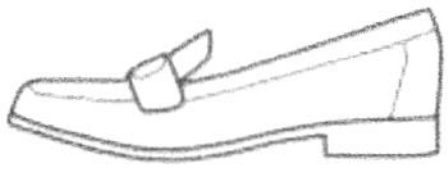

Oxfords

Shoes with closed lacing (the laces go through the upper).

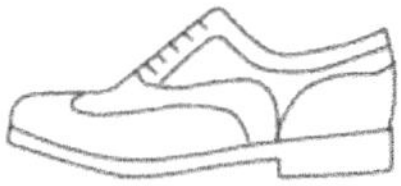

Derbys

A near cousin of Oxfords, the difference is in the lacing: here the lacing is open (the laces go through flaps that can be raised).

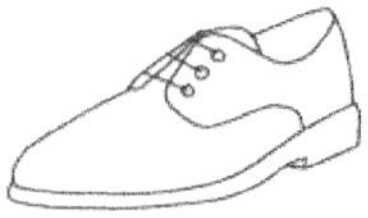

Booties

They cover the feet more than pumps but still stop at the ankle (the malleolus bones).

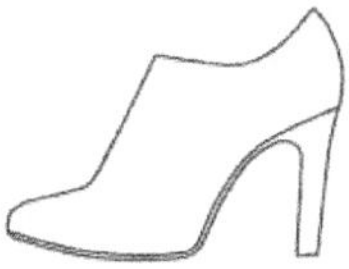

Mid-calf boots

Mid-calf boots vary in height depending on the model, but end somewhere between the ankle and the middle of the calf.

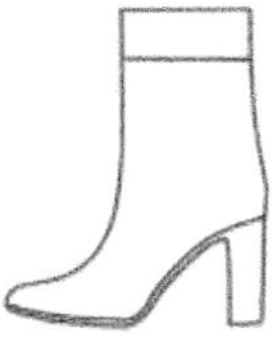

Chelsea Boots

These boots are recognizable for the tab of fabric on the back of the boots and the elastic side panels.

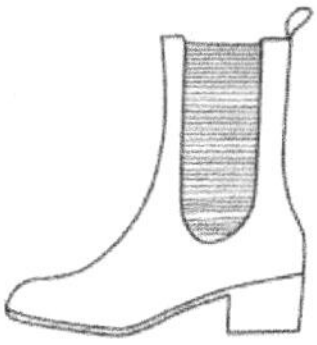

Knee-high Boots

These boots come up to the knee (on or just below).

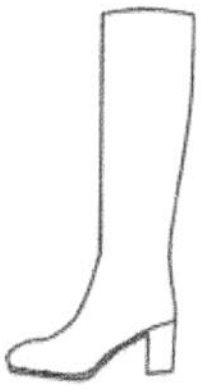

Thigh-high boots

Higher than knee boots, they also cover a part of the thigh.

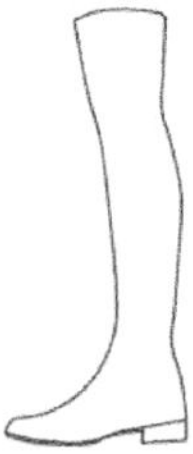

Round toe

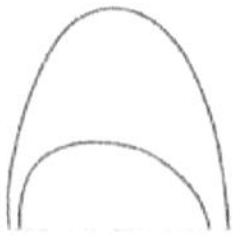

Square toe

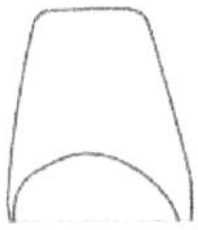

Pointed toe

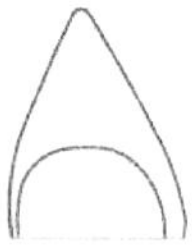

Open toe or Peep toe

There are two different terms for toe openings: peep-toe (a small opening that reveals the big toe) and open-toe (a larger opening that reveals all the toes).

Peep-Toe

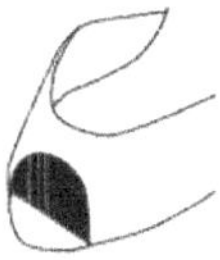

Open-Toe

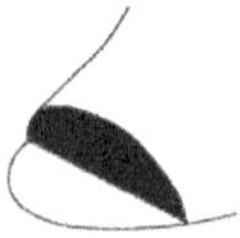

Heels, Health, and Tips

"High heels bring more pleasure than pain."

Christian Louboutin

- Chapter 6 -
The Body and High Heels

The effect of high heels on your body

Although it is best to walk on mid-high heels (1-2 inches), some specialists recommend not exceeding 3 inch heels, except for special occasions (a wedding, a night out, etc.). Despite all the precautions taken, very high heels can be damaging for your body, especially your back and feet.

Wearing high heels enhances your butt (because it arches your back), sculpts your calves, and makes your legs look longer. But that's not all! High heels, especially stilettos, can cause a whole series of side effects. All your weight is shifted onto your metatarsals, more specifically the metatarsophalangeal joints, and your center of gravity is also shifted forward. To compensate, your knees and hips flex, which then affects your legs and your thoracic and lumbar spine. Every part of the body can be affected by wearing heels, from your lumbar vertebrae down to your toes. Some examples? Fractures, sprains, and strains, long term musculo-skeletal problems due to the increased pressure on the muscles and tendons (the shortening of the calf muscles and Achilles tendons), and frequent impact and rubbing (osteoarthritis, arthritis...).

The back, hips, and pelvis

Because the body is pushed forward when we wear high heels, we try to compensate by arching our backs, which then damages the cervical, thoracic and lumbar spine.

When we are in a position equivalent to that of being on tiptoe, the curve of the back becomes more pronounced, and the pelvis is tilted forward, causing lower back pain, and possibly even aggravating an existing sciatica or spine issue.

When we wear heels, the hip hyperextends in order to stay straight and upright. People with osteoarthritis (even in the beginning stages), however, tend to flex their legs.

If you wear stilettos, you should ideally have strong abdominal muscles. There are 3 kinds of abdominal muscles:

- the rectus abdominus muscles: the ones that men build to show off their “six packs”;
- the obliques (external and internal): these are the muscles that allow the rotation and bending movement of the trunk and keep it stable. Situated on the front and side of the abdomen, they play a more important role than the rectus abdominus muscles in flattening the abdomen;
- the transverse abdominus muscles: the two muscles around the lower part of the trunk (cough and you will feel them) that hold the stomach and intestines in place. These muscles can be worked with core muscle strengthening exercises.

Note: the spine continues to grow until a girl is 18 years old. If you are under 18, it is particularly harmful to wear high heels (unless occasional). Be patient!

The knees:

The permanent flexion of the knees when wearing high heels is harmful for people with osteoarthritis of the knees, as it creates excess pressure between the kneecaps and the femurs.

When you wear high-heeled shoes, your feet can't absorb all the impact and so some of the shock reaches your knees (and also your hips). You should therefore be particularly careful if you have osteoarthritis or arthritis, or if you are "at risk".

The calf muscles:

Regular or daily wearing of high heels can cause the gastrocnemius muscles (calf muscles) to shorten, eventually making it too painful to walk without heels.

Moreover, to compensate for the fact that the body weight is shifted forward, the calves remain contracted, causing pain and cramps.

The Achilles tendons:

As with the calf muscles, the Achilles tendons may contract when high heels are worn regularly.

The ankles:

When the weight distribution of your body is shifted, your balance becomes precarious. One of the first joints to try to compensate for this imbalance is your ankles. This causes a significant increase in sprains and strains.

It is therefore important to strengthen your ankle muscles.

The foot:

The higher the talus bone in relation to the tarsus, the more the body weight is transferred to the front of the foot. But the toe and metatarsus bones are not anatomically designed to withstand such a heavy load.

When you slip your foot into a pair of heels, the weight is transferred to a small area at the front of the foot (the metatarsus). This can cause metatarsalgia (synonymous with pain, stinging or burning sensations, and shooting pain if you have Morton's neuroma).

Because all your weight is on the metatarsals, it can also cause hallux valgus (or bunions), as well as pinched nerves in the front of the foot, problems with the foot arch, and degenerative joint diseases of the foot. Bunions can also then lead to a deformity of the toes, known as "hammer toe".

The skin of the foot can also be affected, leading to corns and other calluses.

Blood circulation:

Because the heel is used less, its action as a "blood pump" is diminished. This then leads to cramps, heavy and swollen legs, burst blood vessels, and even varicose veins.

Wearing high (or very high) heels causes an increase in the number of falls, especially in young women aged 20 to 30. The number of injuries due to wearing heels has almost doubled in the United States in the last 10 years. Be especially careful at home, because most accidents take place around the house, when you're paying less attention.

The key lies in moderation. We all love dizzying heels, but you should only wear them from time to time. As soon as you get back home or arrive at your workplace, take them off. When you are traveling long distances, wear low shoes and swap them once you reach your meeting, party, or workplace...

The different shapes of foot and arch

All feet are different, and it is important to identify the shape of yours so you can choose shoes that suit your foot type.

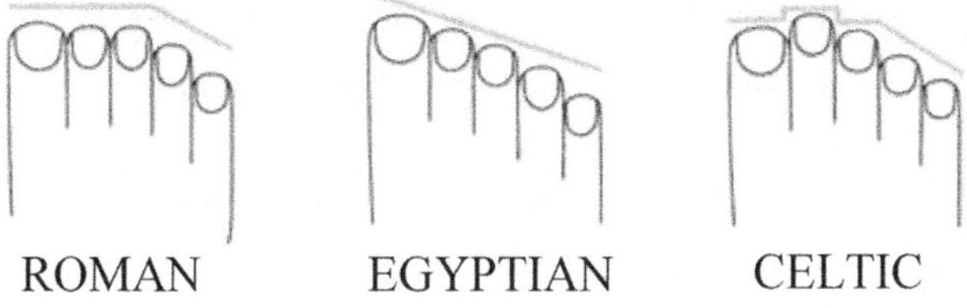

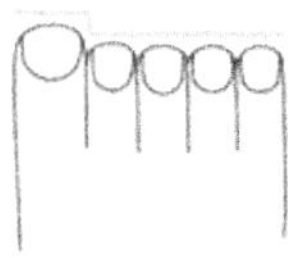

GERMANIC

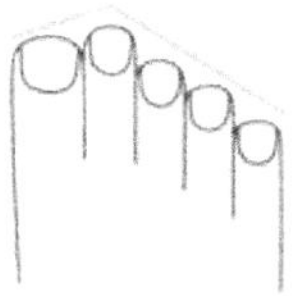

GREEK

For example, a person with Roman or Germanic feet should try to wear round or square ended shoes rather than pointed ones.

There are several different foot shapes. Here are the main ones:

- **Egyptian** feet: the toes decrease in size on a slope (about 2/3 of the population have this foot type);
- **Greek** feet: the second toe is longer than the big toe (about 1/3 of the population);
- **Roman** feet: the toes, especially the first ones, are almost the same length (less common: 6 people out of 100);
- **Celtic** feet: the second toe is longer than the big toe, while the third toe and big toe are about the same length;
- **Germanic** feet: the big toe is longer than the other four, which are all nearly identical in length;
- **Ancestral** feet: although not shown in the diagram, ancestral feet have a big toe that is separate from the other toes, which is particularly the case with bunions.

You also need to consider the arch of your feet. The following diagram (a little exaggerated) will help you identify your arch type.

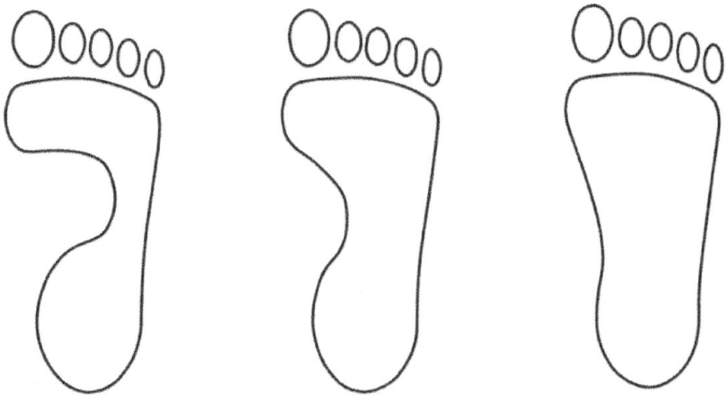

HIGH ARCH NORMAL ARCH FLAT ARCH

The "healthy" arch type is the middle one, where the arch is present, but not too pronounced. If you have a high arch, it can affect your blood circulation: the surface in contact with the ground is not large enough to massage the soles of your feet and encourage the blood to return to your heart well.

Flat feet can cause joint problems (the ankles tip inward, which eventually damages the knees). A podiatrist can make orthopedic insoles to help you. You can also try strengthening your foot (and your ankle) muscles with classical dance or yoga.

What heel height should you choose?

The height of your heels changes (to a greater or lesser degree) the way you hold yourself, which can affect your health.

To begin with, it is important to understand the distribution of your weight on your feet. When your weight distribution changes, it can lead to a large number of health issues.

When you take a step...

> ...with bare feet: 57% of your weight is on your heels and 43% on your metatarsals;
> ...in 1-2 inch heels, the distribution is reversed: 43% of your weight is on your heels and 57% on your metatarsals;
> ...in 2-4 inch heels: 25% of your weight is on your heels and 75% on your metatarsals;
> ...in over 4 inch heels: 10% of your weight is on your heels and 90% on your metatarsals.

Flat to 1 inch heels

- Your feet are comfortable and it is easy to walk, without the risk of losing your balance or twisting an ankle.
- The arch of your foot is not supported.

1-2 inch heels

- The heels begin to lengthen the leg (a little), but are still easy to walk in (especially if the heels are about an inch wide).

- As you get older, they are the best heels for stylish shoes that are easy to walk in.
- Doctors usually recommend heels that are 1–1.5 inches in height.

2-4 inch heels

- You figure looks taller and slimmer, as though your legs go on forever.
- Unless you strengthen your abdominal muscles well and tuck your pelvis under slightly, the heels will change the arch of your back and emphasize your butt.
- If you wear high heels for a large part of your life, your calves will begin to shorten, which will make it difficult or painful for you to wear flat or low heels.
- The risk of health issues associated with wearing high heels (lower back pain, metatarsalgia, bunions, etc.) is higher if you wear them frequently and they are over 4 inches in height. Heels of this height are the most damaging to your body.
- Walking is more difficult, and it is harder to maintain your balance. Which means you are more at risk of falls and sprains...

- Chapter 7 -
The Main Kinds of Foot Injury and Disease

Blisters

Blisters are caused by the repeated rubbing of fabric or leather on your skin. To begin with, the skin reddens. Then, if the rubbing persists, a blister forms, filled with a liquid that protects the skin underneath.

What can you do about them?

❖ *In prevention:*

- To begin with, try not to worry about it... Sounds silly, but it's true. Try sticking silicone patches in your shoes and using hydrocolloid dressings to protect your feet.
- You can apply the moisturizing balm in the recipe in Chapter 11 or use an anti-chafing cream such as Nok Akileine® cream, which is rich in shea butter and is popular among athletes because it prepares the feet for repeated friction. Whichever you choose, massage your feet with the balm or cream, allow it to penetrate, and then put your shoes on once your feet are dry.

❖ *In treatment:*

- If the damage is already done, unless it is so severe that it hurts you, do not pierce the blister. The liquid between the layers of skin will help your skin recover and will prevent the area from becoming infected.
- If you do decide to pierce the blister, do it with a sterilized needle and don't forget to disinfect it well afterwards and then apply a hydrocolloid dressing.
- If possible, avoid putting a Band-Aid on the blister to allow it to dry.
- A dancer's technique? Brush the blister (pierced or not) twice a day with yellow Betadine® for 3–4 days (be careful around your clothes and carpets as it can stain).

Corns and calluses

Corns and calluses are toughened areas of skin on the toes or the soles of the feet due to repeated and prolonged friction. Corns are rounded bumps that often appear dry or discolored, while calluses are flat areas of thickened skin. Although they are benign, corns and calluses can cause real discomfort when walking and a lot of pain (when the core reaches the nerve endings). They can even become infected to the point of requiring surgery.

What can you do about them?

❖ *In prevention:*

- Avoid wearing shoes that are too tight, which can cause corns and calluses.
- Remember to protect areas that rub.

❖ *In treatment:*

- Don't try to "cut off" a corn yourself. You may injure yourself and create infection, without it actually improving the problem.
- You can try corn dressings, such as Compeed® or Scholl® dressings.
- The best solution is to make an appointment with a chiropodist to "treat" your corn or callus.
- Don't hesitate to show your corn or callus to your doctor, especially if you are older and/or have any of the following conditions: blood circulation disorders or diabetes.

Cracks

Cracks are found on dry heels and can be unsightly and sometimes painful.

What can you do about them?

❖ *In prevention:*

- Avoid walking barefoot, especially on rough

surfaces.

- Moisturize your feet as often as the rest of your body.
- Be especially careful in the summertime as wearing flip flops and other kinds of sandals can damage your heels.

❖ In treatment:

- Remove thickened skin with a pumice stone or an electric foot pumice (this must be carried out on dry skin!). I strongly advise against using chemical abrasion creams which tend to overheat the skin.
- Then generously apply a moisturizing cream, like the one described in chapter 11.
- You can also buy creams from the major brands, but rather than using a very synthetic cream, choose one based on active moisturizing ingredients, such as shea butter and oil, argan oil, or cocoa butter.
- If none of this works, consult a chiropodist.

Hallux valgus or bunions

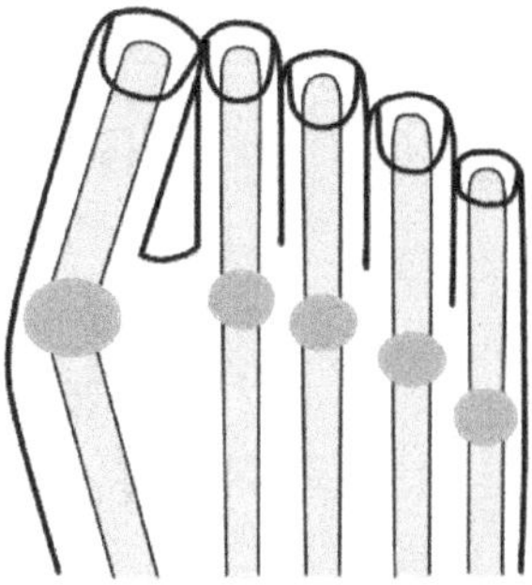

Normally the five metatarsal bones that extend from your toes to the middle of your foot are parallel with each other. In the case of a bunion, the joint connection is deformed, and the first metatarsal moves away from the others, while the big toe is pushed inward toward the other four. This leads the foot to widen at the joints of the toes, causing severe pain and difficulty wearing shoes. Bunions can occur with age or following repeated trauma (wearing pointe shoes for ballet or very high heels in the city for example).

What can you do about them?

❖ In prevention:

- Avoid wearing very high heels too often, especially if the shoe has a pointed tip.
- If you wear pointe shoes (ballet shoes that allow you to dance on the tips of your toes) or closed high-heeled shoes, you can "tighten" your joints by using inch-wide strips that you can find at drugstores to strap them. *(Be careful not to over tighten or you could cut off your blood circulation.)*

❖ In treatment:

- Devices that "straighten" the foot don't help and

can even damage your joints further.

- The only way to fully resolve the problem is with surgical treatment by an orthopedic surgeon. After the operation, however, you will need to be careful not to cause trauma to your foot again. If you don't know which surgeon to choose, find one who operates on dancers... But shhh, that's a secret...

Metatarsalgia

Metatarsalgia is an inflammatory pain felt in the metatarsal area (the metatarsophalangeal joint). It is not serious but the burning sensation can be disabling when you walk or stand on your feet.

What can you do about it?

❖ In prevention:

- Avoid wearing high heels too often, especially if the tips of the shoes are narrow or you are overweight.
- You can put a silicone half-insole under the front of your foot in your high-heeled shoes to absorb the impact a little.

❖ In treatment:

- Start by removing the causes of metatarsalgia described in the "*In prevention*" section.
- Applying a green clay poultice to the soles of your feet can help if you leave it on overnight. (Don't

forget to cover your feet with cling wrap so you don't smear clay about your bed.)

- Consult a chiropodist or even a rheumatologist, who will be able to advise you on wearing orthopedic insoles, doing physiotherapy or osteopathy, taking pain killers, and in the case of unbearable pain, taking corticosteroids.
- Some women on feeling the first pains of a metatarsalgia ask their doctor to do them... a *loub-job* (derived from the name of the famous designer, Christian Louboutin). This involves an injection of collagen or hyaluronic acid on the underside of the foot around the metatarsophalangeal joint, so they no longer feel the pain for a certain period of time, while still wearing stilettos. Of course, this has no protective or preventive effect against the other problems that can affect your feet, such as hammer toe, bunions, etc.

Fungal infections

A fungal infection may appear between your toes, or around your toe nails (making them split), caused by fungi or parasites that tend to develop in humid environments.

What can you do about them?

❖ *In prevention:*

- Try to make sure you keep your feet dry as much as possible, and avoid putting shoes or socks directly on wet feet.
- Try to wear socks made from 100% cotton or other natural materials.
- You can sprinkle the "risk" areas with baking soda before putting on your socks or tights, or even directly your shoes, to absorb any moisture (the bicarbonate of soda will also reduce any unpleasant smells).

❖ *In treatment:*

- You can do a foot bath with baking soda: dilute 4 tablespoons of baking soda in 4 cups of warm water. Let your feet soak for 15 minutes before taking them out and drying them thoroughly.
- Locally, you can dab the affected areas three times a day with cotton dipped in a few drops of the following mixture: 25 drops of essential lavender oil and 22 drops of essential tea tree oil mixed with 2 teaspoons of quality vegetable oil (first cold-pressed olive oil or argan oil). Repeat for 3 weeks.
- If the situation doesn't improve, see your doctor.

Morton's neuroma

This condition is characterized by intense pain. It is caused by wearing high heels with narrow tips which leads to a thickening of the tissues around a nerve that is found between the 3rd and 4th toe.

What can you do about it?

❖ *In prevention:*

- Never, or only occasionally, wear stilettos with pointed toes.

❖ *In treatment:*

- There is only one solution: surgery.

Ingrown toenails

An ingrown toenail is a nail that has grown into the skin because it is too long or has been cut too short at the corners, or due to wearing very tight shoes. It can lead to inflammation and pain. If nothing is done, the area may become infected.

What can you do about it?

❖ *In prevention:*

- Take care of your feet: avoid letting your nails grow too long or cutting them too short at the corners.
- Avoid wearing shoes that are too tight.

❖ *In treatment:*

- Before the situation gets worse, make an appointment with your chiropodist.
- Otherwise you will need surgery.

Plantar warts

A plantar wart (verruca) is caused by a virus, the human papillomavirus (HPV). Plantar warts can develop if you have an immunity deficiency, even temporary, or damaged and/or wet feet (for example a cut on the foot). You will notice you are infected, because the area becomes painful or because you can see a surface of rough skin with small black dots on it.

What can you do about them?

❖ *In prevention:*

- Avoid walking bare foot in public places, especially humid places (campground showers, public swimming pools, etc.).

❖ *In treatment:*

- Because of the risk of infecting those around you, even though some verrucas disappear on their own, I would advise you to treat them as quickly as possible.

- You can apply a salicylic acid solution (available in drugstores) for one month. Or you can try cryotherapy, where the wart is burned at about -400°F with liquid nitrogen (at home or by a dermatologist).
- Although plantar warts are benign at the start, if you let them develop, you will have no choice but to go through surgery (again!).

- Chapter 8 -
How to Choose your Shoes well

Here is some advice when choosing a new pair of shoes:

1) Try the shoes you want to buy at the end of the day rather than in the morning. That way, while your feet are more swollen, you can choose comfortable shoes that won't hurt your feet by the end of the morning. Avoid shopping after a very long, hot day on your feet however: once your feet have cooled down again, you will find that your feet are lost in your new shoes. I won't give the example of a woman who spent a summer's day dashing about the shopping malls in Milan, Italy and who bought a beautiful pair of pumps at the end of the day, only to realize the next day they were a size too big. No, it's not worth insisting, I won't mention that example.

2) Choose shoes that you find comfortable to wear. Suffering will not make you more beautiful. If there is a pair you really like but that hurt your feet too much, you can always buy the shoes and put them on display in your home. After all, some shoes are real works of art.

3) Choose a shape adapted to the curve of your foot, and try to buy shoes with shanks (the supportive structures under the soles that gives them their arch). Metal shanks are more durable than plastic shanks, giving your shoes a longer life (they will collapse less quickly).

4) When trying on shoes, always walk with both feet in the same pair of shoes (some people like to try a new shoe on each foot from two different pairs). If they hurt too much in the store, there is little chance it will improve over time.

5) Rather than buying several pairs of bad quality shoes, invest in a good pair of shoes that will last.

6) If you are a little overweight, choose a thick or wedge heel rather than stilettos. Not only will thin heels make you unstable, but they will make your legs look wider than they really are.

7) Make sure the heel is well centered so you don't lose your balance. For this, you need to try them, but you should also look at them. Is the heel too far back? Or does it come slightly forward as well as being centered at the top? (Shoes like this are the most stable.) You are a glamorous woman, not a ninepin!

8) If you can't decide about a pair, don't buy them! If you really find them that beautiful and comfortable to wear, the

choice should be an easy one! But not being able to decide is a choice in itself...

- Chapter 9 -
Learning to Walk in Heels

Walking in high heels makes us look more confident and sensual. Provided you know how to walk in them. You can too learn to walk with poise and sex appeal. Here are some tips...

Strengthen your abdominal muscles and look taller

As we saw in the chapter about the effect of wearing high heels on your body, your back can particularly suffer. You should try to keep your abdominal muscles strong and squeeze your butt a little so that you don't arch your back too much. At first you will need to remind yourself regularly, but it will gradually become a habit. *To help you tone your abdominal muscles, go to the 3rd part of this book.*

Hold your head straight, as though there is a string pulling you up from the top of your head. Your chin should be neither too low nor too high, and your shoulders relaxed.

To keep your balance, lean your upper body backward slightly and tilt your pelvis under.

Some women get into the habit of sticking their butt out to keep their balance and leaning their upper body forward. To counter this, they then have to flex their knees more than is necessary. The posture described above avoids this! Yes Mademoiselle! You're wearing pumps, not ski boots. And the only slippery slope around here is in running up your credit card bill at the shopping mall!

Look straight ahead of you

High heels can make you look cool and confident, so long as you're not spending all your time looking your feet. Yes, I know it can sometimes be hard not to do when you're having to watch out for dog poop on the sidewalks, or dodgc around drain covers, which is never easy in high heels.

When you walk, lift your chin and look into the distance ahead of you. Your step will become lighter, and you will look like a model sauntering by, far above the base material considerations that affect ordinary mortals. You are worth so much more than that! At least that's what people will think!

Make sure you keep your eyes fixed on a point in the distance (like when you drive a car) as this will help you maintain your center of balance. Walking like a baby giraffe is not for you!

If possible, choose comfortable shoes

There is nothing more unsightly than a woman with sore feet. You can tell a woman's feet are sore by the way she walks. She'll look like she's hopping from one foot to the other, to avoid being in contact with the ground for too long. Or her face will be tense, her jaw clenched, and her lips pinched.

Some luxury shoemakers believe that a quality shoe should be pleasant to wear. Don't forget what Manolo Blahnik once said: *"There is nothing charming about a woman who can't walk in her shoes."*

But this isn't always the case. Some pumps are just so beautiful, that you simply *cannot* do without them. Even if they do torture your feet. In that case, you need to use all the tips and tricks in this manual to reduce the pain: creams, silicone patches, salves... Bear in mind too that wedge heels are your friends, even if they are high.

Relax and stand tall

Unless your boyfriend is C-3PO, robotic walking is just not for you. Relax! It will make you look more graceful and feminine.

You can soften your hips and knees to help you, or swing your arms slightly to accompany your movement (and help you keep your balance). Think of bracelets that jingle softly to the rhythm of your step. *Note: keeping your knees soft doesn't mean you have to bend them.*

Start small

If you're used to wearing flat shoes or low heels, don't suddenly start wearing very high heels overnight.

Begin by wearing shoes with thin little heels, such as 2 inch kitten heels. Then move on to 3 inch heels and keep getting higher if you would like to end up wearing a magnificent pair of 4 inch stilettos.

Little journeys

Practice! Walking with high heels is not natural, and it will take several days or even weeks for your body to get used to walking at a new height.

It's not a good idea to wear your heels for the first time when you're about to go out partying with your girlfriends, on a shopping spree, or spending the day tramping about the corridors at work.

Begin by wearing them at home: it's time to wear your shoes in. This will help avoid blisters due to the stiffness of the leather, and it will also give you the chance to see if any seams rub and to put a gel patch on them... Another test for you to try out: the staircase. Sooner or later, you're going to be confronted by a flight of stairs. So start by practicing at home or in the stairwell of your building. When you climb upstairs, only put your toes down. When you go downstairs, put your whole foot down (toes and heel at the same time). The railing can be of precious aid, and can even be glamorous if you let your fingers slide over it without clinging on too tight.

Once your shoes fit comfortably on your feet, only go out in them for short journeys and small trips that don't last long: to fetch your suit from the dry cleaners or your bread from the local bakery, for example.

The easiest is to take something with you that you can support yourself on (a trolley or your little nephew or niece's stroller), and to gradually test out your balance by walking back and forth among the supermarket aisles, doing little turns and pivots, moving from one foot to the other...

Put your heel down first and then your toes

Put your heel down first, then your toes, and finally shift your weight onto the tip of your toes before taking another step. You want to walk as naturally as possible, while being careful not to drop your heel down too heavily onto the ground (you don't want to make too much noise while walking: your heels should tap on the ground, not hammer it).

If you want to imitate the likes of Gisèle Bündchen, try walking down an imaginary line, one foot in front of the other. This will make your legs cross in front of each other and your hips sway. But be careful: you should really master your balance before doing this. (Have you ever noticed the number of models that fall over during fashion shows?)

To walk more lightly, turn the tips of your toes outward slightly without spreading your legs: they should be no more than hip width apart.

Adapt the length of your step

There are two different theories on this. Try them both and use one or the other according to your need: looking seductive or walking fast.

The first: the higher your heels, the shorter the length of your steps. Don't try to take longer strides, or you will end up bending your knees, which will give you an unattractive, jerky look.

The second: the longer your strides without unrolling your foot, the more stable you will be. You will be able to walk faster, but is it really attractive? It's up to you to decide: at the end of the film *The Devil wears Prada*, watch Anne Hathaway walking in the streets of New York after making a last phone call to Meryl Streep. Practical, yes. Glamourous? It's your call.

Do regular stretches throughout the day

Wearing high heels all day puts pressure on your body. In this book you will find some easy stretches to incorporate into your day. Pay particular attention to your ankles, calves and lumbar vertebrae. *Go to the 3rd part of the book.*

Look after your feet and shoes

To reduce aches and strains and reward your feet for carrying you about all day long, pamper them with foot baths, pedicures, and repairing creams. There are tips and tricks on this in the following chapters.

Changing your shoes each day gives your feet a rest (the arch and heel differ from one pair to another, as do the areas where the seams may rub), and it also lets your shoes recover, giving the leather the chance to air and to dry if your feet perspire, which then extends the life of your shoes (and reduces unpleasant smells).

Avoid wearing heels when pregnant

As pregnancy advances, a woman's stomach grows (and her back arches) pulling her center of gravity forward.

Wearing high heels will make this worse. That is why it is more difficult for a pregnant woman to stay balanced in heels, and it can become dangerous, as she is at more risk of falling.

Wear low to medium heels (1-2 inches) if you are pregnant. Avoid thin heels and wear wedge shoes which distribute your weight more evenly.

- Chapter 10 -
Tips and Tricks

How to make your shoes more comfortable

More and more brands are making accessories that you can insert into your shoes: patches, insoles, half-insoles, and heel protectors, made of gel or foam, in different colors, for closed or open shoes, non-slip, shock absorbent… there's something for everyone.

When you buy new shoes, wear them at home for an hour or two (stroll about a bit, don't stay sitting on the sofa) so you can see if they rub or hurt anywhere and sort it out as quickly as possible!

To avoid blisters and burns due to repeated rubbing, you can also put talc in your shoes if you wear them barefoot (the talc will absorb any perspiration) or use baking soda (which will also reduce unpleasant smells). There is another old home remedy that involves rubbing the inside of your shoes with dry soap, but you may not go that far…

How to make your shoes bigger

There are three different solutions:

- If you have leather shoes, you can run them under hot water, then quickly put them on and keep them on until they dry. The leather is softer when warm and will mold to the shape of your feet. But you will need to put up with wearing wet shoes for a while... The risk? While some types of leather respond well, others may not like it so much.
- You can buy a special shoe stretch spray designed to help enlarge your shoes. Spray it inside and outside your shoes in the toe area. Then put your shoes on and keep them on for a while.
- You can also put shoe trees in your shoes as soon as you take them off. Some people use shoe stretch spray just before putting in the shoe trees.

These techniques can help you gain half a size or mold your shoes to fit your feet. Of course, the best option is obviously to buy shoes that fit your feet in the first place. You can also take your shoes along to a cobblers but if you've tried the solutions presented here and they haven't worked, you may find yourself footing a bill at the cobblers' for nothing.

How to make your shoes smaller

Buy a magic wand and ask Hermione Granger for help. No, seriously... You just can't shrink a pair of shoes.

On the other hand, if you have a pair of shoes that are too big, there are some tricks you can use so your feet aren't lost in them (which will also help reduce any rubbing). The first option is to stuff cotton into the tips of the shoes. If you find that too makeshift, you can take them to the cobblers, where they will fit a kind of half-insole, which they will trim to the size needed. And once it's been fitted, it won't move anymore!

How to avoid damaging your feet too much (and the rest of your body)

Once your shoes are ready to wear, remove them as often as possible: when you arrive home, when you sit down at your desk...

Only put them on just before you reach your workplace or appointment, and do most of your journey in ballerina shoes or derbies, for example.

Avoid wearing heels more than 2 days a week.

How to sprint in heels

For starters, if you need to get sprinting, make sure your shoes don't slip. Then, pick up speed by setting down just the tip of your toes and not your heels. You can only run for a few hundred meters like this though, or your calves will give in...

How to make sure you never get caught out

When choosing the shoes you're going to be wearing for the day, ask yourself, *"Where am I going to be walking?"* in other words *"What kind of surfaces will I be walking on?"*

Putting on a pair of stiletto heels to go to the park where they might sink in the ground? Bad idea. Wearing your patent pumps on gravel paths? Not so great. And how are you going to manage to walk about on cobbled paving? Walking lightly on the tips of your toes (unless you're wearing wedge heels).

What other option do you have? The one I mentioned earlier. I repeat: do most of your journey in flat shoes or low heels.

Caution: Unless you have a spare pair of shoes in your handbag, never take your shoes off far from your car or home because they're hurting too much or you won't be able to put them back on again after!

How to drive in heels

It's not a good idea to drive in shoes with a flat heel: you'll end up damaging the heel counter (the back of your heels tends to rub the floor of the car when you press down on the pedals).

But driving with very high-heels is not a good idea either because you'll tire yourself out for nothing!

The best option is to leave a pair of comfortable old shoes or sneakers under the driver's seat. When you climb in or out of the car, you can just swap them. And *voilà*… you're all set to go!

How to make sure your feet don't slip about in your shoes

When women wear high heels, the pain is often concentrated around the metatarsophalangeal joints (the joint between your toes and the rest of your foot). This is experienced as a burning sensation on the pad of the foot, due to the fact that the front of the foot has to support a large part of your weight (which it's not made for).

To ease the pain, you can buy silicone half-insoles to put in the front of your shoe. This will make your shoes more comfortable and reduce the burning sensation.

The pain can also be made worse if your foot slips down and is "crushed" into the bottom of your shoe. In this case, you can take some hair spray and spray it onto the insole around the arch of the foot. This will help you to "grip on" inside the shoe.

How to avoid slipping over

Some people recommend wearing the same pair of shoes often when you go out, because the more you walk in them, the more the soles will become scuffed and less slippery. Not only does this technique not necessarily work (some heels are still just as slippery after several hours' walking outdoors), but you may also wind up on your back like a beetle on a gusty day.

I have a couple of "safer" tips:

- Score the soles of your shoes (for high-heeled shoes, only score the toe end) with a few short strokes of a scissor blade or a cutter, or sand them with a sheet of sandpaper.
- You can also take your shoes to a cobblers' who will fit them with a non-slip sole.

If you are a fan of the famous shoes with red soles, you will notice that as with many luxury and/or high quality shoes, the soles are made of leather. This makes them extremely slippery at first, and then the soles quickly become scuffed. Some may exclaim, "Yes, but I don't want to ruin my shoes!" or "I don't want to change the color of the soles! They have to stay red!" In this case, you can take them along to your local cobblers and see if they can fit a non-slip red sole. Alternatively, you can take your shoes to Minuit Moins 7, passage Véro-Dodat in Paris. This cobbler holds the exclusive rights for repairing and fitting Louboutin soles. And if you aren't planning a trip to Paris? No fear, ladies! You can send your favorite pair by post! I recommend you use registered post. (If you live in London, you can take them to Minuit Moins 7 in Whitecross Street, n°163–165.)

How to find a good cobbler

If you don't whether your local cobbler has a good reputation, start by leaving them a pair of shoes that don't have too much financial or sentimental value to you, rather than leaving them your best pair of Ferragamo stilettos.

Did they do a good job? Well that's great news. Was their work shoddy? Well at least you didn't let them get their hands on your favorite pair of pumps.

How to take care of your shoes

Before you put them on for the first time, waterproof your shoes with a product designed for the purpose. You can buy protective sprays at a cobblers or at the supermarket.

Keep them clean. Even the most beautiful pair of ankle boots can look shabby if they are covered in dirt or dust. You can scrub them with a soft brush to get rid of the worst of the dirt, then use a special shoe cleansing lotion on a piece of cotton. (There are soft rubber brushes especially designed for suede, or you can remove the worst of the dirt by gently scraping it with your nail and then rubbing it with a white stationery eraser.)

Don't wear the same pair of shoes two days in a row, to give them a chance to air and dry (especially if you tend to perspire).

Be careful when storing them (don't throw them on top of each other), and when putting them on (using a shoehorn may seem old fashioned, but it helps avoid crushing the heel counter or damaging your manicure). Finally, don't leave them in a room that is too damp, hot, or in direct sunlight.

How to relax your feet after a long day

Sit up straight on a chair (or relax back on the sofa...) and place a tennis ball or yoga ball under the sole of one of your feet. Roll the ball backwards and forwards under your foot, then make small circular movements for 5 minutes. Then switch to the other foot. This technique will relax your feet, encourage blood circulation, and reduce swelling.

You can also use a wooden massage abacus. Set it down on the ground, and while you are sitting, roll your feet back and forth over it for about ten minutes. This technique will help you relax and stimulate your blood circulation, just like with the tennis ball technique.

In the evening (and also in the morning), you can also run the soles of your feet under a jet of water at 60°F / 15°C (hydro-massage position) to relax your feet and encourage blood circulation. You can continue by running the jet of cold water over your legs moving upwards from the feet to loosen them up and prepare them for the day ahead.

- Chapter 11 -
Recipes you can make at home

When you buy your supplies, choose ingredients that have been grown with organic farming, biodynamic agriculture, or the regulated harvesting of wild plants. Because taking care of Nature is the first step in taking care of yourself.

Seeing that some of my recipes are for using in the bath, some people may exclaim, *"Shock horror! That's not very environmentally friendly all that!"* In response to these people: polluting the planet and wasting drinking water don't concern us here. In developed countries, the water is very efficiently collected and treated. The recipes below are all based on natural ingredients and are therefore biodegradable. Don't feel guilty if you sometimes take baths with water that is easily treated. The problems of water pollution concern industry more than individuals who use essential oils and other natural products. And besides, if it's to take a twenty minute shower...

Caution and warnings:

- To avoid overdosing, don't use all these recipes on the same day.
- Respect the recommended doses.

- Even if some essential oils can be used by women when pregnant or breastfeeding, as a precautionary measure, I would advise against using any of the recipes that contain them.
- The following recipes and the products used in them are intended for adults only and <u>not for children</u>, for external use only. In addition, the following recipes and the products used in them should be kept out of reach of children.
- If you are unsure whether any of the products used are harmful to you in any way, consult your doctor or pharmacist. They alone are qualified to advise you.
- By continuing to read the cosmetic recipes described below, you acknowledge that you are fully aware of the list of precautions for use and counter-indications set out in the appendix at the end of this book, that you are aware that this list is not exhaustive, and that only your own full and total liability may be incurred if you decide to make these cosmetic recipes or use them. In no case may the liability of the author, the illustrator; or the publisher be incurred; and for any use of the natural products described in the following recipes (powders, hydrosols, essential oils, vegetable butters and oils, etc.) for therapeutic purposes, you should consult a doctor or a recognized health professional.

Before making your own cosmetic recipe:

- Do a skin test (as described in the appendix).
- Disinfect all the containers and utensils you are going to use.
- Wash your hands thoroughly and/or put on disposable gloves. Then put on an apron, a dust mask, and safety glasses, and tie back your hair or put on a hair net.
- Be careful to avoid burns and splashes when heating the products to add to your recipes.
- Store your recipes in a cool place and use them relatively quickly after making them. If you ever notice that the texture, color, or smell etc. of your recipe has undergone the slightest change, throw it away with your household waste.
- Don't forget to label each of your recipes with the name of the preparation and the date of manufacture. Then, store your recipes and the products used to make them out of the sight and reach of children.

Recipe 1: Effervescent foot bath balls

These effervescent bath balls are wonderful for relieving your feet after a long day. Just drop one into a tub of hot water.

They will soothe and repair the damage your shoes have done to your skin thanks to the healing action of the kpangnan butter and avocado oil. The bay leaves also have a cleansing action, and the lemongrass and the pink peppercorn stimulate blood circulation.

Baking soda	60 grams
Citric acid	35 grams
Kpangnan butter	30 grams
Avocado vegetable oil	10 grams
Bay leaf vegetable oil	10 grams
Lemongrass essential oil	70 drops
Pink peppercorn essential oil	45 drops

Mix the baking soda and citric acid in a bowl and then set aside.

Using a set of kitchen scales, put the Kpangnan butter in a bowl, then melt in a bain-marie and remove from the heat. (Please note that you should only "*melt*" and not "*cook*" the butter). Add the avocado oil and bay leaf oil, and mix.

Combine the two mixtures. Then incorporate the lemongrass essential oil. Mix. Add the pink peppercorn essential oil. Mix.

The mixture will froth and crackle. Put it in the freezer for 5 minutes, then take out the dough and shape it into small balls (or other shapes if you prefer). Put in the fridge for several hours until the balls harden.

These effervescent bath balls can be stored for up to 2 months if you keep them in an airtight box in the fridge.

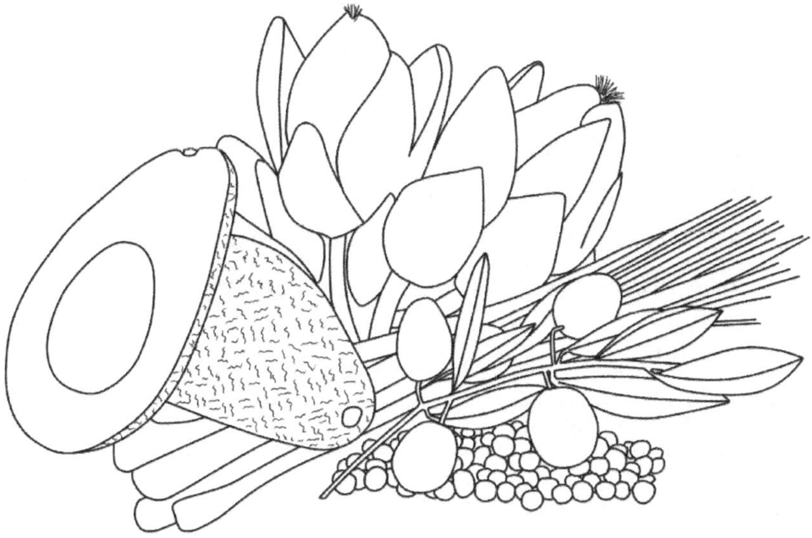

Recipe 2: Refreshing anti-perspirant spray

This spray will really refresh your feet. Thanks to its essential oils, it also relieves swelling and works as an antiperspirant.

You can pour 10 ml of the mixture described below into a small spray bottle and keep it with you in your handbag. If you keep it in the fridge, this spray will be even more cooling for hot feet on a summer's day.

The peppermint hydrosol has tonifying and refreshing properties, and can help reduce excess perspiration. This effect is enhanced by the clary sage and Mediterranean cypress. The rose geranium is antiseptic and antifungal and is useful in preventing fungi from developing on damp feet. Solubol is a natural dispersant that helps incorporate essential oils (fatty substances) in an aqueous solution. *Note for sensitive noses: the smell is quite powerful.*

In a 125 ml bottle:

Peppermint hydrosol	100 ml
Solubol	240 drops
Clary sage essential oil	55 drops
Mediterranean cypress essential oil	30 drops
Rose geranium essential oil	20 drops

Combine the solubol and the three essential oils. Once the solution is evenly mixed, pour in the peppermint hydrosol and stir.

Pour the mixture into a spray bottle and use to spray your feet once or twice a day, as needed, or systematically every morning and evening for a short period.

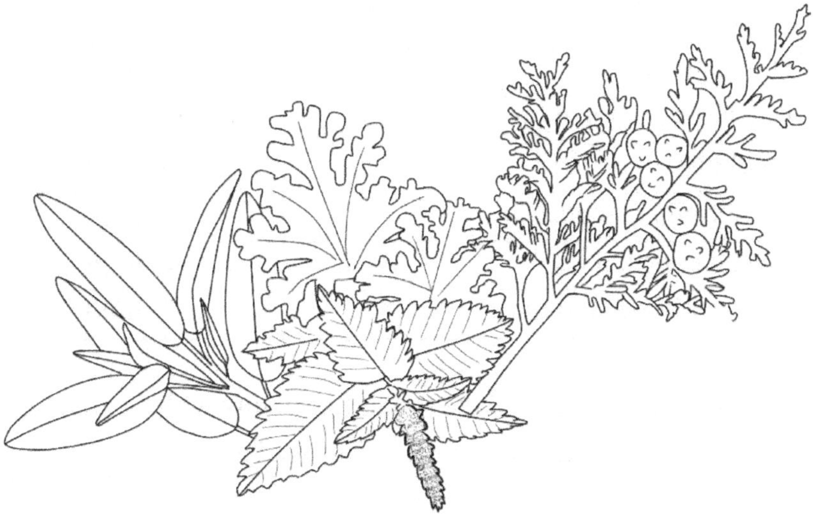

Recipe 3: Circulatory gel

This cooling gel can be applied to your legs (and why not your feet too) to relieve the sensation of heavy legs and promote blood circulation. Apply this gel morning and night to reduce swelling.

The little bonus? This gel dries very fast and will moisturize your skin, leaving it feeling silky smooth. For an even fresher effect, keep the gel in the fridge.

For a 100 ml bottle:

Pure aloe vera gel	85 ml
Butcher's broom extract	220 drops or 10 ml
Solubol	160 drops
Peppermint essential oil	40 drops
Mastic essential oil	32 drops
Grapefruit seed extract	21 drops

Dilute the essential oils in the solubol, then mix with the aloe vera, butcher's broom extract, and grapefruit seed extract.

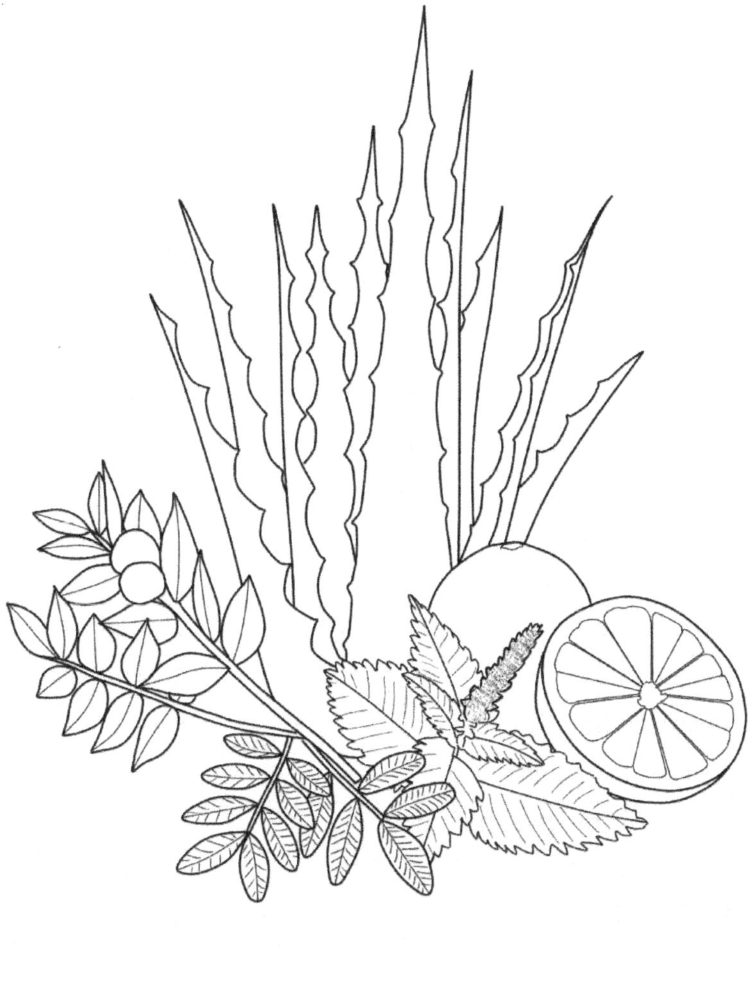

Recipe 4: Moisturizing balm

This moisturizing balm will deeply nourish your skin. Apply to your feet up to the ankles (insist on the heels and the pads of the feet, as well as your toe nails if they are brittle), massage in, and then leave to dry. Goodbye dry, cracked heels! You can also apply this balm to your legs and elbows...

The two vegetable butters are wonderful for their nutritional and moisturizing properties, and the kokum butter doesn't leave a greasy film on the skin. The tea seed vegetable oil is great for dry skin and brittle nails. The jasmine wax and essential oils will give your balm a sublime and sensual fragrance. Finally, the vitamin E will act as a natural preservative.

In a 250 ml container:

Kokum butter	100 ml
Shea butter	100 ml
Jasmine Grandiflorum wax	8 grams
Tea seed vegetable oil	16 ml
Ylang-Ylang essential oil	30 drops
Neroli essential oil	26 drops
Vitamin E	12 drops

In a bain marie over low heat combine 100 ml of kokum butter with 100 ml of shea butter, and 8 grams of jasmine grandiflorum wax.

Once the mixture has melted, remove it from the heat. Wait until it has cooled down and is luke warm.

Add the camellia vegetable oil, the essential oils, and the vitamin E. Mix thoroughly until completely smooth and even.

Transfer to an airtight container and allow to cool at room temperature until the mixture is firmer to the touch (and white).

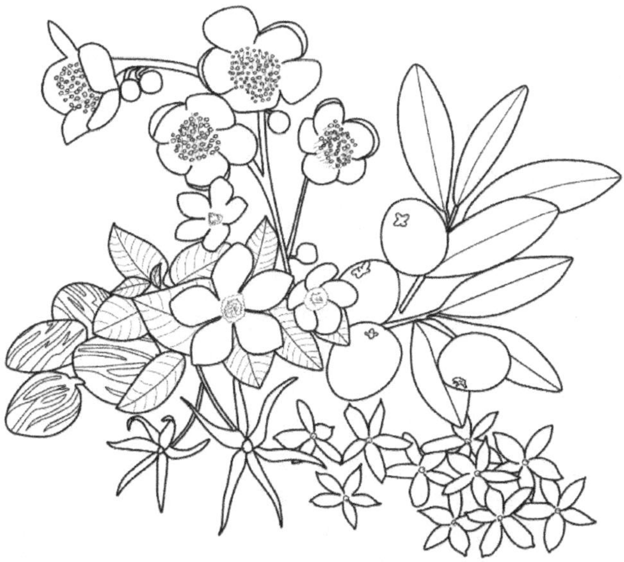

Recipe 5: Healing body bath

After a long day on your feet, you can have an aching back, stiff shoulders, and swollen legs. From time to time, it is good to take a moment to pamper yourself and look after your body. Slip into a nice hot bath with a glass of wine in one hand and a magazine in the other.

This recipe will help relieve contractures and tone your microcirculation:

Epsom salt	140 grams
Pomegranate CO_2 extract	44 drops
Katafray essential oil	62 drops
Lavandin Super essential oil	58 drops
Virginia Cedarwood essential oil	34 drops

Combine all the ingredients in a bowl. Mix thoroughly, then store these bath salts in an airtight container.

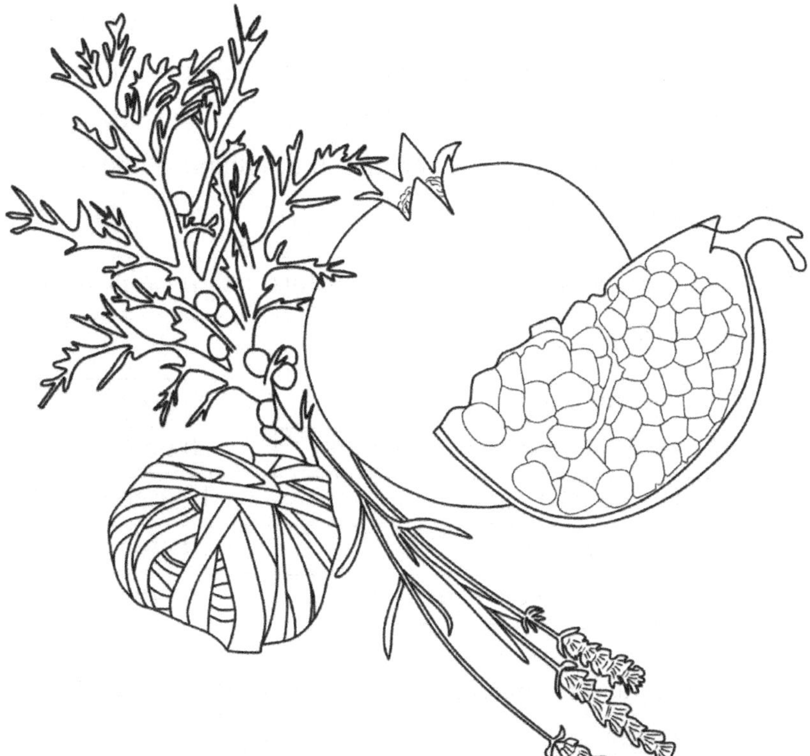

Recipe 6: "Goodbye Crocodile Skin" bath powder

Ideal for irritated skin and eczema, this pampering bath powder will soothe and repair your skin, leaving it all soft. Perfumed with damask rose, it helps to relax and unwind.

Centella asiatica is a plant that regenerates the skin by stimulating the production of collagen, while the sweet almond milk powder nourishes the upper layers of the epidermis. The allantoin and honey powder are used to enhance the softening and repairing properties of the bath powder.

When you run a bath, pour a little of this bath powder under the running water:

Sweet almond milk powder	60 grams
Damask rose powder	20 grams
Honey powder	10 grams
Allantoin powder	10 grams
Centella asiatica powder	10 grams

Incorporate all the ingredients in a bowl. Stir thoroughly until evenly mixed.

This bath powder will keep for six months in an airtight container.

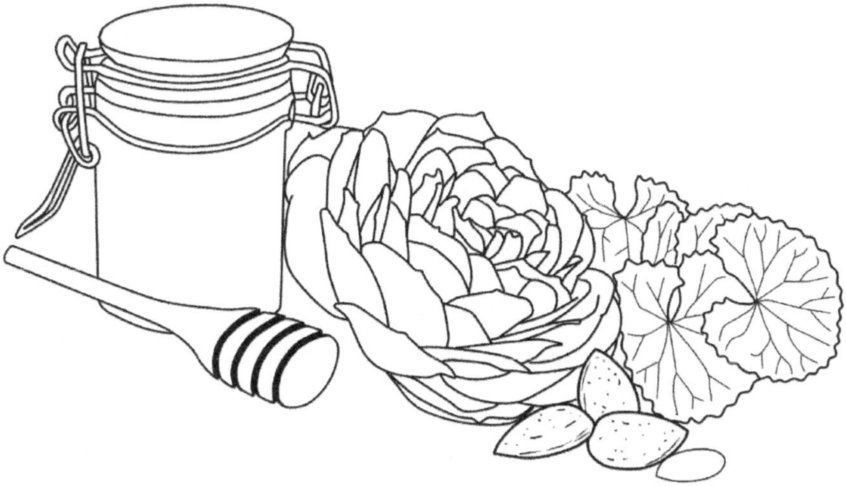

- Chapter 12 -
A Home Pedicure

It is important to take care of your feet. If not simply because you think they deserve it (after all, they carry you about all day long), then for health reasons. Healthy feet suffer from less pain and injury and are better able to withstand uncomfortable shoes.

If you're still not convinced, then imagine you twist your ankle in the middle of the street. A valiant knight who looks the spitting image of your favorite actor comes to your rescue. And you're going to laugh, but it just so happens he's an orthopedic surgeon! (I know, what are the chances…) He wants to check your ankle, so he kneels down beside you. You feel the warmth of his left hand as it delicately cups your ankle. Then he gently slides off your pump with his right hand. And there... He finds himself faced with a foot fit for an ogre! Are you really tempted by this scenario? So do the following once a week...

1) Take off your nail polish with nail polish remover.

2) Rub any corns or calluses (thick, hard skin, especially common on the heels and pads of the feet) with a pumice stone or foot file.

3) Soak your feet for 5 to 10 minutes in a basin containing warm water, lemon juice, and a handful of coarse salt. (This will help you clean around your nails.)

4) Take your feet out of the water and dry them well with a towel.

5) Use a little boxwood stick (available in department stores) to push back the softened cuticles around your nails. (Never cut your cuticles as they act as a tight seal between your nail and your skin, blocking the bacteria.)

6) Using nail scissors, or better still nail clippers, trim your nails. Don't cut them too short (it's not attractive and it can be painful), and don't leave them too long either (they could break against the end of your shoes). To reduce the risk of ingrown toenails, don't cut too far down the sides of your nails either (giving them a square or rectangular shape) by slightly rounding the corners.

7) File the edges of your nails to prevent them from getting caught. If you ever notice streaks or little "waves" on the surface of your nails, polish them.

8) Apply a nourishing foot cream to your feet and ankles, and massage them a little. (You should moisturize your feet daily.)

9) If you would like to wear nail polish, first paint a base layer to protect the nails, then apply a double layer of polish. To make the polish more resistant you can apply a top coat. If you've gone over the edges of your nails, wait until your polish is dry and then rub with a cotton swab dipped in nail polish remover.

Tone, Strengthen, and Stretch!

"Wearing your dreams on your feet, is the first step in making your dreams become reality."

Roger Vivier

- Chapter 13 -
What you Should Know before Starting...

We are now going to look at some exercises you can practice to strengthen, tone, and stretch the different parts of your body you use when wearing high heels.

For this, we are going to use techniques from different disciplines that are known to both strengthen and stretch the muscles: yoga, classical dance (in particular, floor barre techniques) and pilates (a practice that was initially developed for classical dancers). You will notice that these different methods involve similar movements, and resemble each other in terms of the benefits they bring and the way they work the body. Don't forget that the yoga poses can also be used for meditation, which isn't the case for the other exercises.

Of course, these exercises and stretches are provided for information purposes only and have no medical intent. Using them does not mean that you shouldn't still consult an osteopath or physiotherapist.

For newcomers to yoga, you should be aware that each pose should be compensated by another. To give you a clearer image: if you bend your torso forward, you should then bend it backwards, and vice versa.

The benefits of each exercise and stretch are described below. Unless any special mention is made, there are no contraindications because the first contraindication is that imposed by your body itself: pain. If the exercise hurts you or you dread the idea of a particular pose, avoid it and listen to your body! This book was designed to help reduce any aches and pains, not to make them worse. If you ever have a doubt about a pose (for example, *"Is the Butterfly Pose bad for my knee?"*), consult a health care professional who knows you well. Every case is different, so it is difficult to go into all the disorders and conditions that a reader could suffer from.

Note:

In order to avoid injury, you must use the correct neutral positions that all the exercises begin with.

The position of your head and neck:

- Imagine a string pulling you up from the top of your head, and your eyes looking straight ahead of you.
- Your chin should not be tilted too far forward or backward.

The position of your shoulders:

- Your shoulders should always be as low as possible, and drawn slightly backwards, to clear the neckline.

The position of the spine:

- When you are lying down, your spine should be in balance: neither too arched nor flat against the ground.
- To find the correct position when you are lying on the ground, you should bend your knees a little. Then, still keeping your spine in the same position, extend your legs. This is the neutral position that your lumbar vertebrae should be in. You should be able to slide a hand underneath the small of your back.

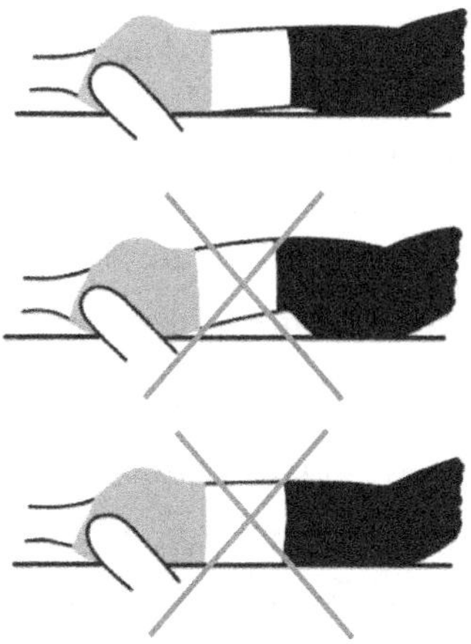

Mountain Pose:

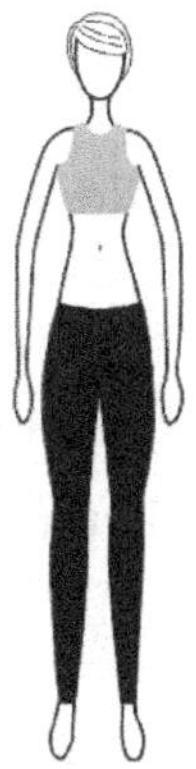

- Stand with your feet hip width apart, your arms by your side, and your shoulders back, looking straight ahead of you, your body relaxed. Your ankles, knees, and hips should all be aligned, and the weight of your body should be spread over the entire surface of your feet.
- This yoga pose ensures you are well grounded and is the starting point for many other poses.

So you can make the most of the static exercises described in this book, I also suggest you use **abdominal breathing**, especially during the yoga poses. It will help you relax, and therefore stretch better, as well as massaging your organs.

To begin with:

- Lie on the floor, in a neutral position, with your legs slightly apart and your shoulders back.
- Place your hands on your abdomen so you can feel the movement better.
- When you inhale: the air enters your lungs and your belly expands, as though your navel is trying to reach the ceiling (be careful not to arch your back!).
- When you exhale: you let out all the air from your lungs and your navel moves back toward your spine.

According to the proper rules of the art, for the yoga exercises you should inhale gently as you count up to 4, hold your breath for 4, then exhale for 4, and finally hold your breath for 4 again. Little by little, you can increase this up to 6, 7, or 8!

Normally, you only inhale and exhale through your nose and not your mouth, in order to warm the air. But if you prefer you can inhale through your nose and exhale through your mouth.

- Chapter 14 -
How to Do a Session

As with any practice, you should start gently and build up gradually. Don't think that just because you are doing dance, pilates, or yoga exercises, there are no risks: an injury can always happen. The most important warning sign is pain: if a movement hurts, stop immediately. If necessary, make an appointment with your doctor, physiotherapist, or osteopath to find out whether the exercises and stretches are appropriate for you.

When you look at an exercise, don't tell yourself, "*I'll never be able to do that!*" The only limits are those you set yourself. Of course, you won't become as flexible as a master yogi overnight, but you can build up, gently and repeatedly.

Wear loose and/or stretchy clothing (a dance, yoga, or jogging outfit for example...) so you can move comfortably, and don't wear shoes (barefoot or socks only).

Even if you only have a few minutes to spare, always do a warm up. Below are just 5 quick warm-up exercises so you can do your practice safely. So why risk doing without them?

If you decide to do muscle strengthening exercises, still do the stretches. Some people may want to skip the "*Exercises*" section though and just focus on the stretches.

At the end of the session, if you like, and if you have the time, you can do a little relaxation exercise.

Note before starting:

1) You can refer to the table at the end of this chapter: it summarizes all the poses, exercises, and parts of the body you will be working. Some stretches, for example, work the same muscles, so choose the ones you feel most comfortable with.

2) You will see the word "Yoga" in brackets beside the names of some of the poses so you know which discipline the exercise comes from. If nothing is written, then the movement comes from classical dance and/or its derivatives (floor barre and pilates).

3) In the descriptions of the exercises, you may sometimes read *"sitting on the ground"* or *"lying on the floor"*. Some people may roll their eyes and say, *"Well I'm not exactly going to lie in the air or sit on a wall!"* But the reason I insist on this, is that you need to be on a hard, flat surface. Otherwise, some people may be tempted to do the exercises sitting or lying on a bed... If you like, the floor exercises can be practiced on a yoga mat or a blanket.

- Chapter 15 -
Warm up

This is an essential step to prepare your body for the exercises that follow and to avoid any injuries. It takes place at the start of a session. Begin by gently working your shoulders, neck, back, arms, and legs. Even if you only want to do the exercises to strengthen your legs, you should still warm up your upper body.

Warm up 1 - The Back, Chest, and Shoulders

Begin by standing with your arms by your side, and your feet hip width apart.

1) Let your hands slide under your butt and roll your upper back and neck forward as you gently bend your knees. You should be aiming to stretch your spine, as though you are creating a space between each vertebra. *Hold the position for 30 seconds.*
2) Keeping your legs parallel and your knees bent, interlace your fingers at your coccyx. Slowly pull yourself upright, trying to bring your elbows as close together as possible (you may even be able to get your elbows to touch). This new position should be accompanied by a movement of the upper back, as though you are trying to get your sternum to face the ceiling. Your head should be tilted slightly backwards. Be careful not to raise your shoulders. You may like to imagine your shoulder blades trying to come together. Feel how your chest opens up and broadens in this position and how your shoulders draw back a little. *Hold the position for 30 seconds.*

Quantity: Slowly and gently repeat this sequence 3 times.

Benefits: This little sequence will help you warm up your back and shoulders and work your neck a little, as well as "opening up" the rib cage.

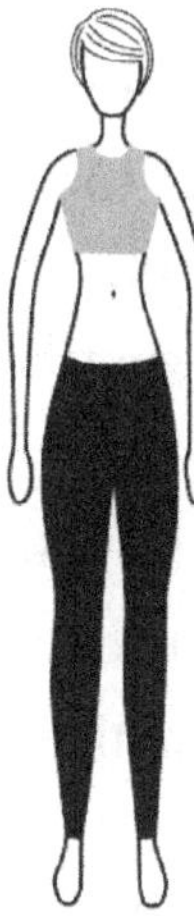

1

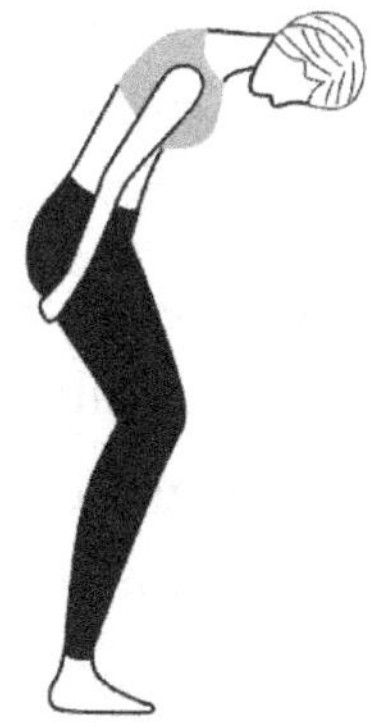

2

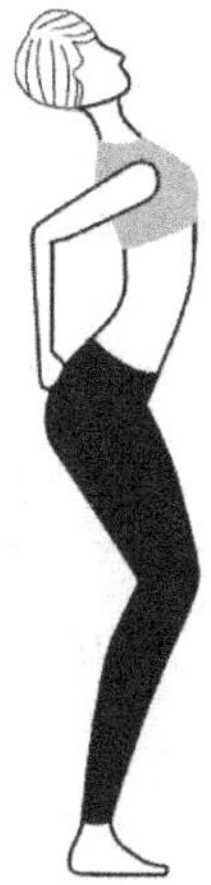

Warm up 2 - The Spine

1) Begin by standing with your arms by your side, your feet parallel and hip width apart, and your knees slightly bent. You should be looking straight ahead of you.
2) Keeping your spine as straight as possible and pushing your ischiums (sit bones) backward, bend your body at the hips until your back is parallel to the ground.
3) From this position, continue downward, rolling your spine from the middle of your back down to your head. You should do this step slowly, trying to notice the movement of each vertebra.
4) To finish, "unfold" yourself, starting with your lower back and ending with your head, imagining you are straightening up vertebra by vertebra.

Quantity: Slowly repeat this sequence 3 times.

Benefits: This sequence will help you warm up and gain awareness of your spine and each of your vertebrae. By pushing your sit bones backward, you will feel your hamstrings stretch.

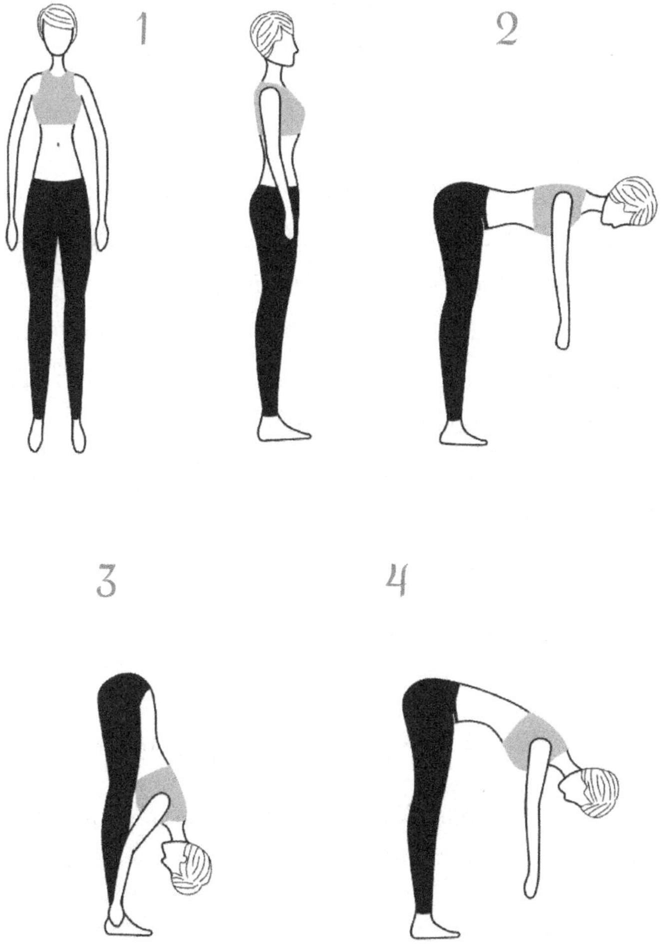
1
2
3
4

Warm up 3 - The Neck

1) Sit cross-legged on the floor. Your head should be straight without your chin being tucked under, your shoulders relaxed, your hands on your knees, and your abdominal muscles engaged.
2) Gently tilt your head to the right, as if you want to touch your right shoulder with your ear. *Hold the position for 10 seconds*. Return to the initial position, then tilt your head toward the left shoulder. *Hold the position for 10 seconds.*
3) Repeat the exercise gently tilting your head forward and then backward. *Hold for a few seconds each time.*
4) Rotate your head from right to left, sweeping the room with your gaze. When you turn your head, your chin should come almost above your shoulder, and your eyes should look as far behind you as possible.

Be careful not to raise your shoulders during this exercise.

Quantity: Repeat steps 2), 3) and 4) five times.

Benefits: The "basic" neck warm up used in gym classes at school.

1

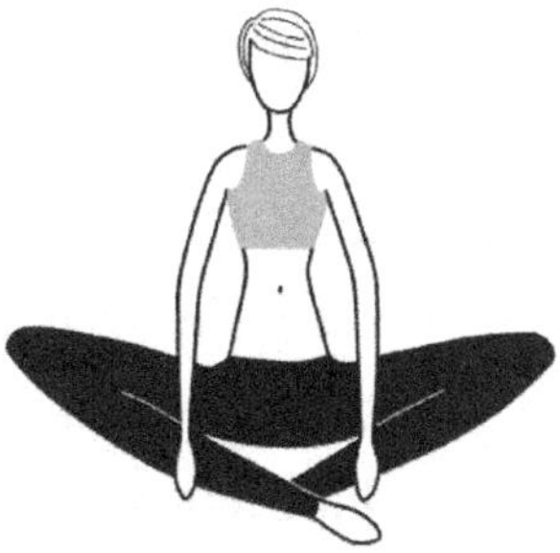

2

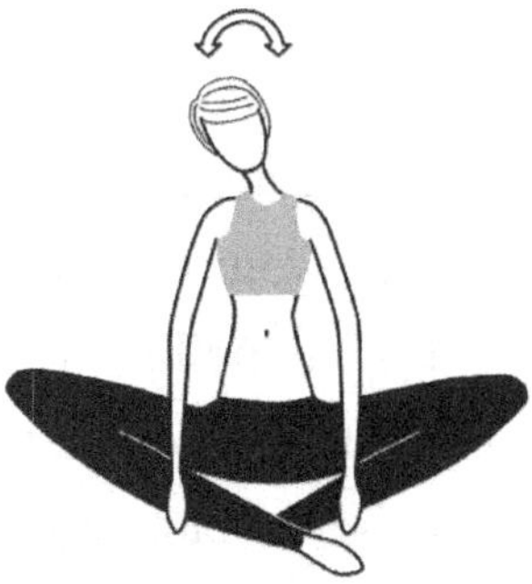

3

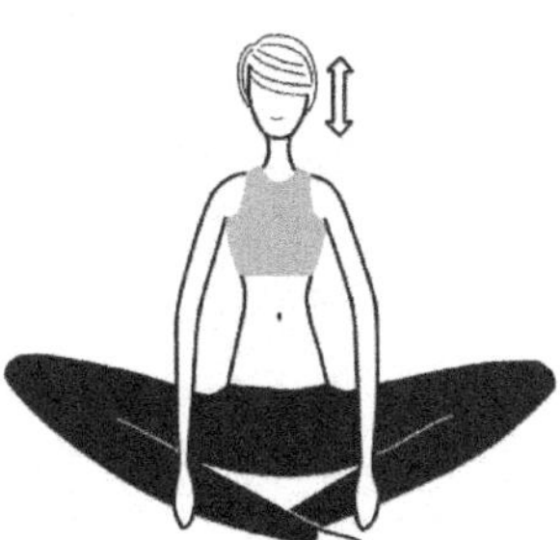

4

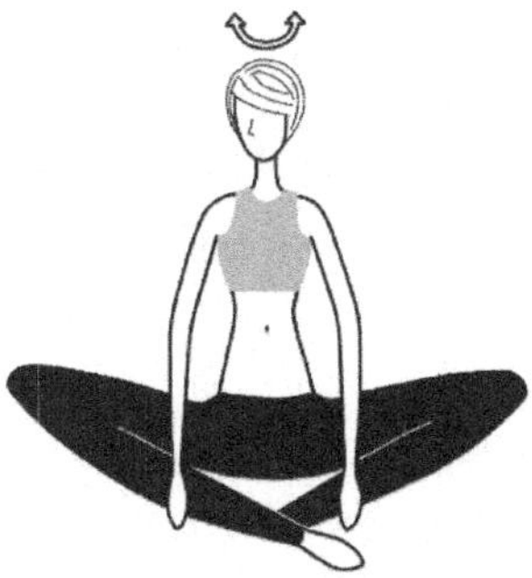

Warm up 4 - The Neck

1) Stand with your feet together, your head and back straight, your arms by your side, and your shoulders relaxed.
2) Take your left elbow in your right hand.
3) Lightly pull your left arm downward with your right hand, while you gently tilt your head to the right. You should feel a light stretch in your left shoulder and the left side of your neck, but it shouldn't be painful.
4) Gently return to the starting position and repeat on the other side. This time, take your right arm with your left hand and pull it downward, while you tilt your head to the left.

Quantity: Slowly tilt your head alternately to each side 10 times.

Benefits: This warm up helps stretch the neck and shoulder muscles and is ideal for relieving tension due to stress.

1

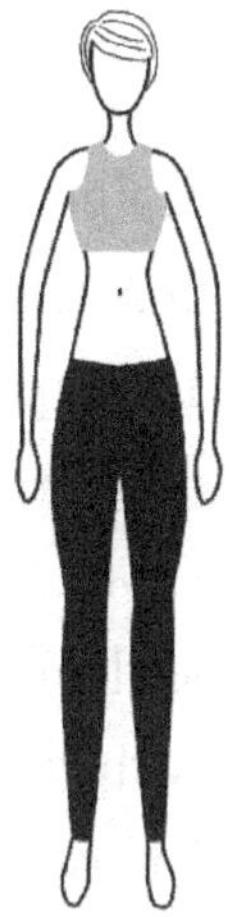

2

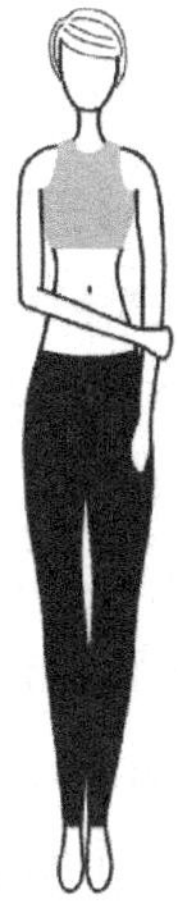

3

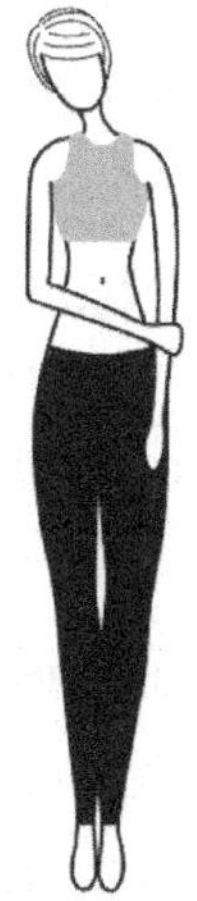

Warm up 5 - The Hips

The hips come under particular pressure when wearing high heels.

1) Lie down on the floor on a towel or yoga mat, with your arms by your side and your legs straight and in line with your hips (your feet should be about a hand width apart).
2) Try to stay relaxed, but remember to keep your abdominal muscles engaged. Your back should be resting on the ground, without being too arched nor completely flat. A little indication: your shoulders, and the top and middle of your spine should be in contact with the floor, but you should still be able to slide a hand between the floor and the small of your back.
3) Now slide one of your hips up toward your head as if you want to "push the joint into your belly", while your other hip slides down toward your feet as if it is going to "come out of its socket". You should do this movement without moving or lifting your butt, which stays on the ground. Seen from above, your pelvis should be oblique.
4) Repeat the movement with the other hip.

Quantity: Repeat the movement 5 times for each hip.

Benefits: This up and down movement stretches the hips and pelvis. As well as loosening it up, it will help you gain awareness of a part of your body that isn't often specifically targeted.

1

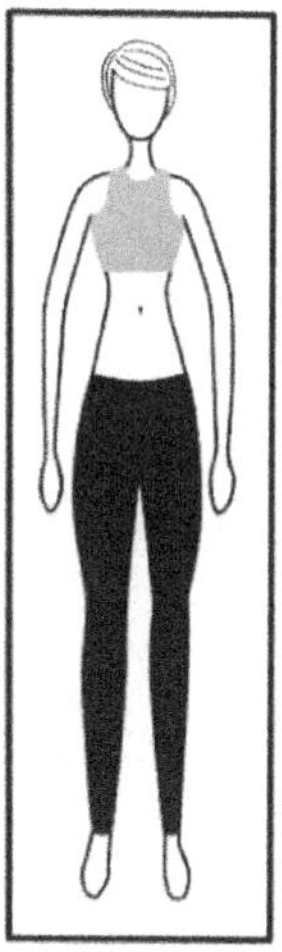

2

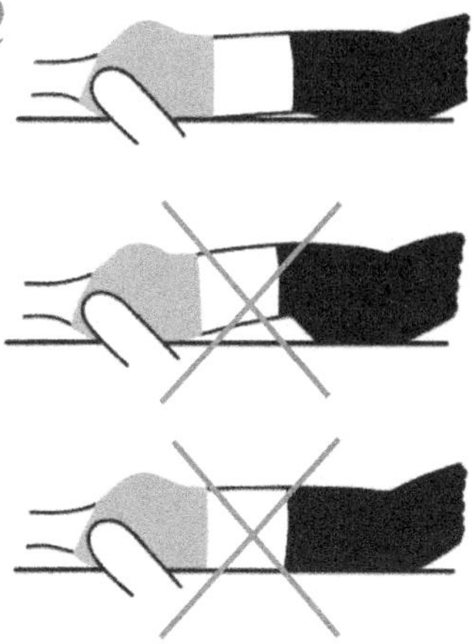

3

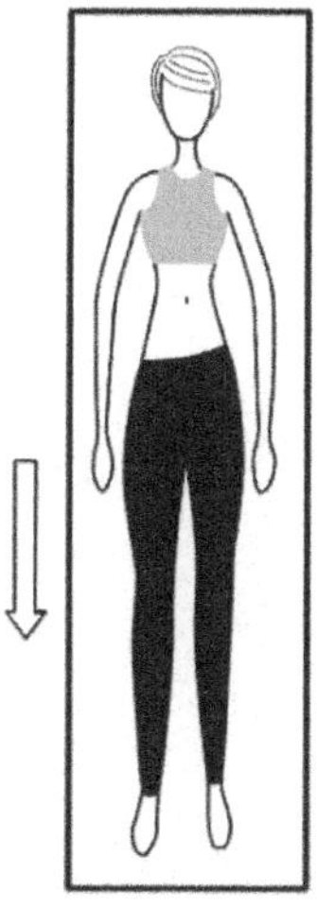

4

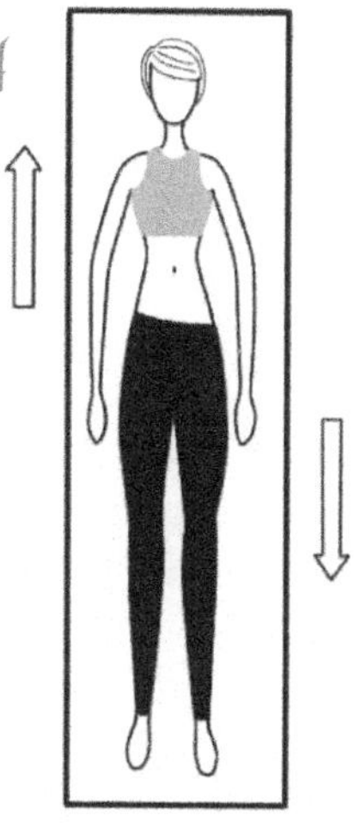

- Chapter 16 -
Exercises

The following exercises are popular with classical dancers and involve a combination of barre exercises, floor barre exercises, and pilates. But don't panic, everyone can do them! If you look at pictures of dancers, you will notice that their bodies are very slim but their muscles are clearly sculpted. The unique thing about dancers' muscles is that they are elongated. You won't see any bodybuilders on stage, and yet they are strong and powerful enough to make prodigious jumps, hold incredible positions, and carry their partners...

This is what we are going to reproduce here: exercises to finely tone your muscles, stretch your limbs, and strengthen your body and joints. Given the subject of this book, we are only going to be looking at the parts of the body affected by wearing high heels. So please be aware that these are not complete floor barre, pilates, or yoga sessions. If you like, you can focus exclusively on exercises that work a specific part of your body, depending on your need. You should try to practice these exercises at least 1 to 3 times a week. But nothing prevents you from doing more than this. Having said that, try to avoid practicing intensively every day for the first week, to then end up only practicing occasionally afterward…

Exercise 1 - The Stairs

This exercise can be done standing up beside a wall, but it is best done on a step so you can stretch your calves as far as possible.

1) Place the front of your feet on the edge of a step and hold on to the railing. Lift one foot. This will force you to transfer all your body weight onto the other leg and work your balance.
2) The railing is there to support you and prevent you from falling, but you shouldn't cling on to it or force down on your arms. You should only be trying to work your lower body. However, you should still be engaging your glutes and abs (so you don't arch your back), as well as the leg you are standing on.
3) Are you well aligned? Most of your weight should be on your heel and not the front of your foot.
4) Now lift your heel as high as you can, as though your body is being pulled up toward the ceiling. *(In classical ballet, it is said that your foot is in a demi-pointe position.)*
5) Then come back down again, trying to extend your leg as far as possible, without hurting yourself, to stretch out the back of your calf.

Quantity: Do 3 sets of 20 foot raises to start with for each leg. Then gradually increase this up to 40.

Benefits: This exercise will help strengthen your calves (the gastrocnemias muscles) and tone the muscles of your feet and ankles. If you can practice it on a step rather than flat on the ground, it will allow you to extend your calf further and stretch out your tendons and other ligaments.

1

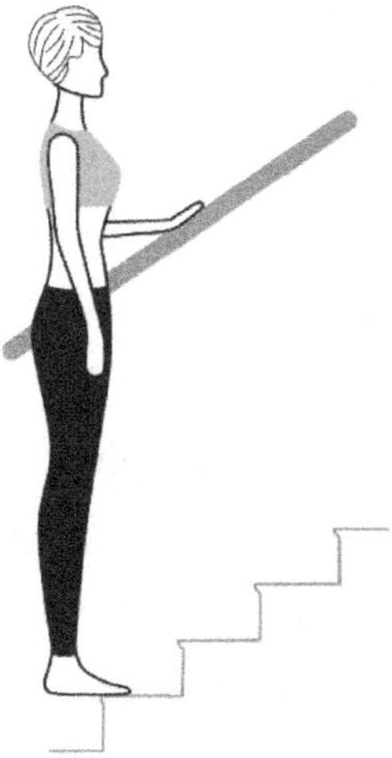

4

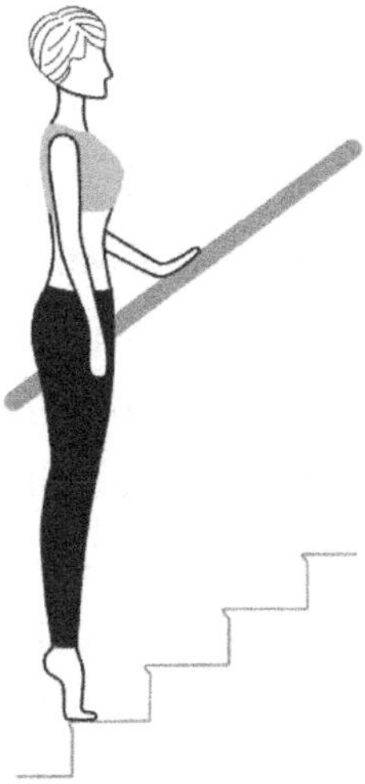

5

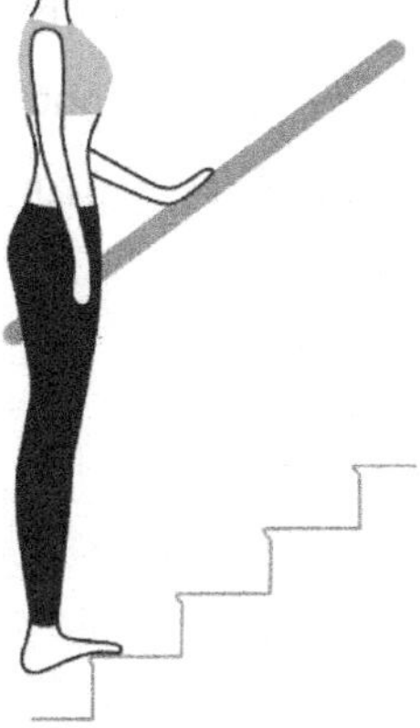

Exercise 2 - Pliés/Relevés

Pliés and relevés can be done standing up, but here we are going to do them the floor barre way.

1) Lie down on the ground in a neutral position. Your head should be aligned with your spine, your eyes looking at the ceiling. Place your hands on your hips. Your legs should be extended and pointing outward (your feet should be turned to the sides), with your heels touching and your feet flat against a wall. (If you know classical dance, put your feet in first position.) *You should keep your abdominal muscles engaged throughout this exercise.*
2) Do a demi-plié: bend both your knees, keeping your heels together. This brings your feet up toward you (your feet should now be where the top of your calves were in position 1). Your knees should be pointing outward and as near the ground as possible.
3) Extend your legs again to move back to position 1).
4) Go up onto a demi-pointe position: your feet should push against the wall until only your toes are in contact with it. Your legs should be straight and firm.
5) You will have moved away from the wall, so move back before starting again.

Quantity: Repeat 3 sets of 6.

Benefits: This sequence of pliés and relevés helps tone the muscles of the feet, ankles, calves, and thighs.

1

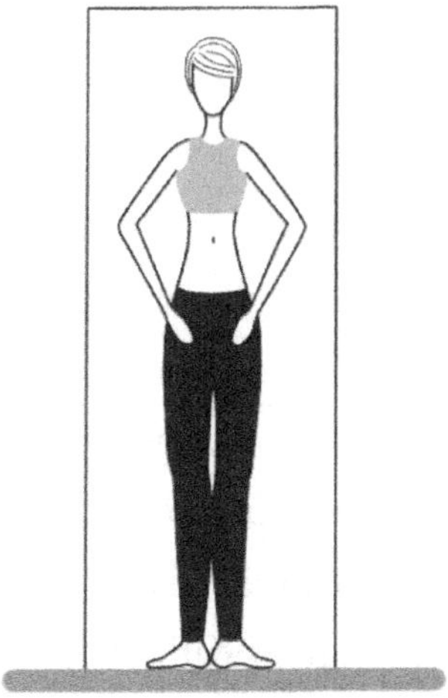

2

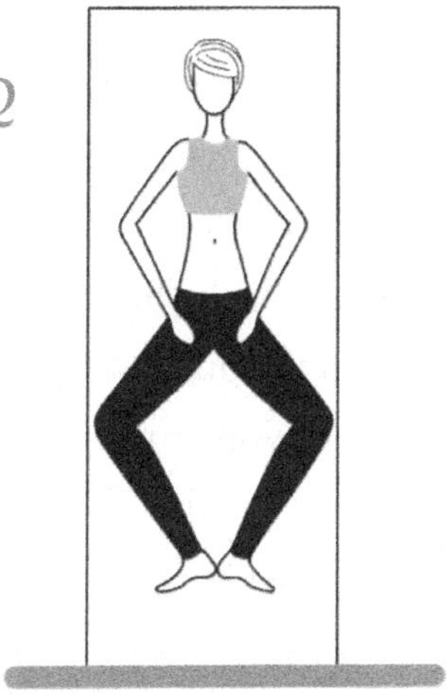

3

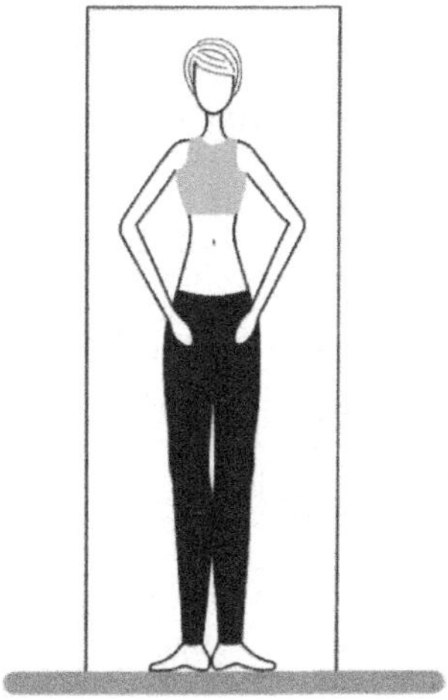

4

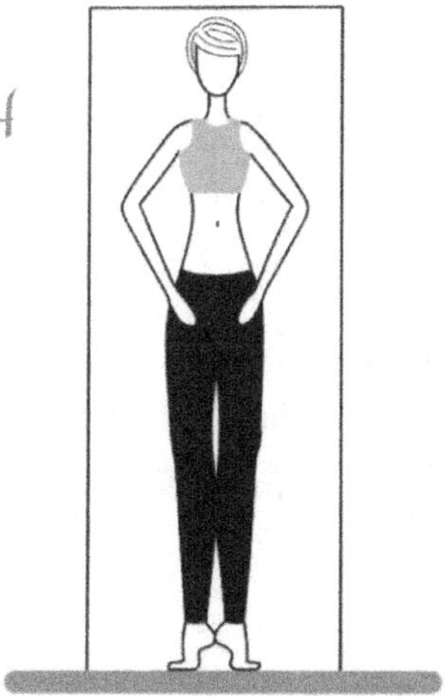

Exercise 3 – The Dragonfly

This exercise is based on the same principle as the butterfly position, but helps tone the thighs and butt.

1) Lie on your back, with your arms by your side, your knees bent, and your heels on the ground.
2) Lift your heels off the floor (and only your heels). Your lower back should become rounded and come into contact with the ground, while your butt lifts upward.
3) Open your legs. For this, imagine someone placing their hands on the inside of your knees and pushing them to either side of your body. The rotation takes place at the hips, while your feet stay in alignment with your tibias.
4) Close your legs until your knees touch. You should be back in position 2.

Note: during this exercise, make sure your lower back stays in contact with the ground at all times, and don't forget that the rotation takes place at the hips.

Quantity: Repeat steps 2) to 4), doing 3 sets of 12 with 15 seconds break between each.

Benefits: Ideal for toning the thighs and butt.

1

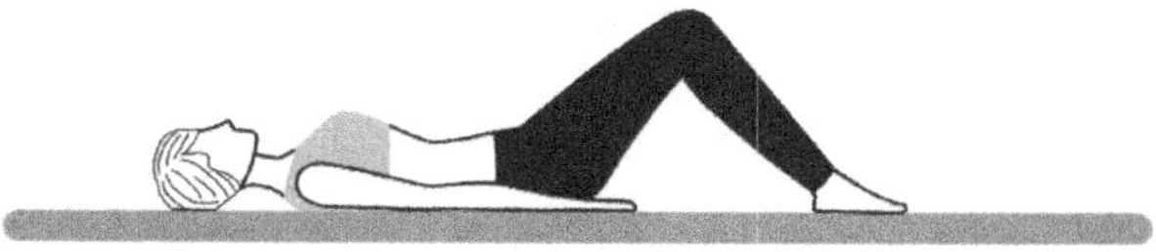

2

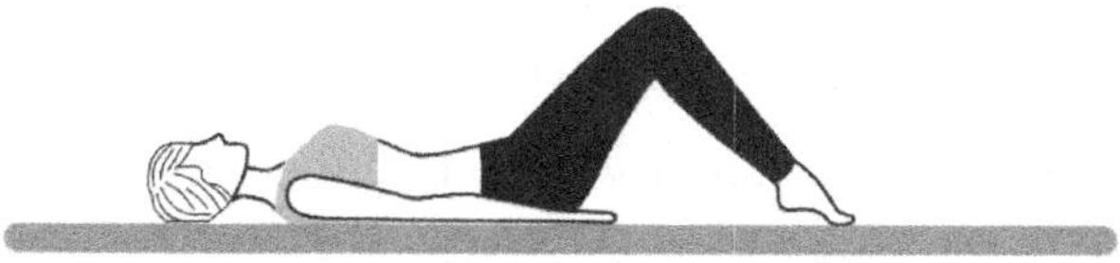

3

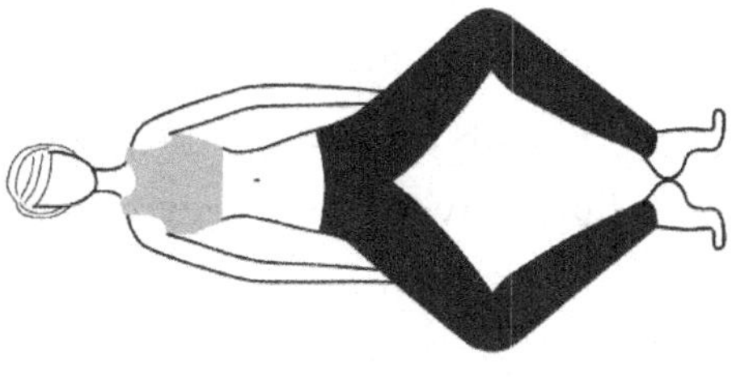

4

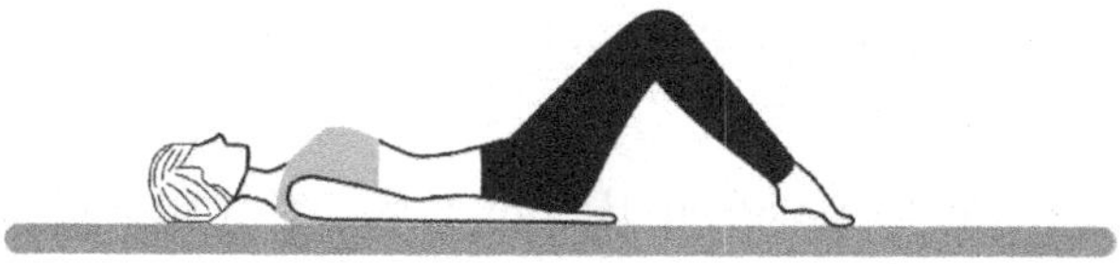

Exercise 4 – The Abdominals and Lower Back: Strengthening, Posture, and Stability

Having strong abdominal muscles helps reduce back problems as well as some digestive disorders. However, working the abs with crunches (lying on the floor, with your legs bent, and lifting your chest up to your thighs) "pushes" your organs down and weakens your pelvic floor. It is better to strengthen your abdominals with static, isometric poses (i.e. by contracting the muscles without any movement), which doesn't force down on your organs.

The three different poses that work the transverse abdominals to give you a flat stomach, from easiest to hardest, are the following:

1) In a plank position, facing the ground, with all your body weight on your hands and toes. From a side view, your back should be aligned with your legs. Your arms and legs should be straight and your triceps and pectorals engaged. You should be looking at the ground below your head.
2) Identical to position A, but you lower yourself down onto your forearms. Your elbows should be under your shoulders, and your forearms and hands should be pointing forward.
3) Identical to position B, but instead of being under your shoulders, your elbows should be slightly forward.

1

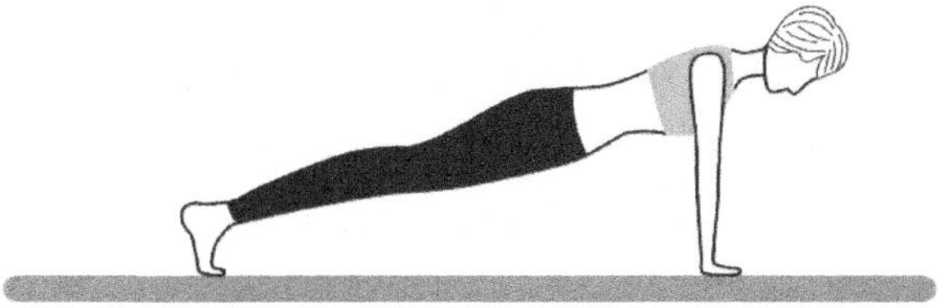

2

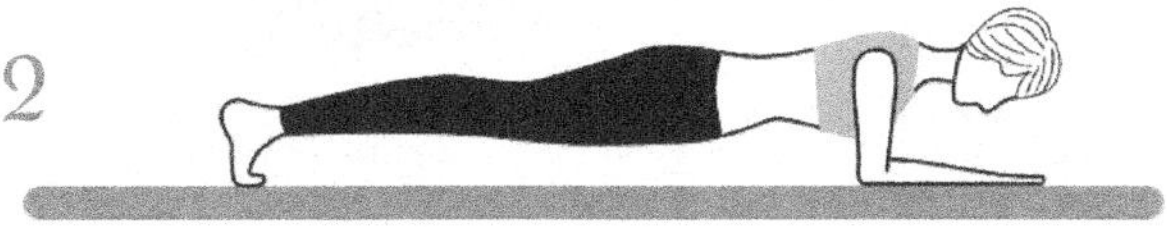

3

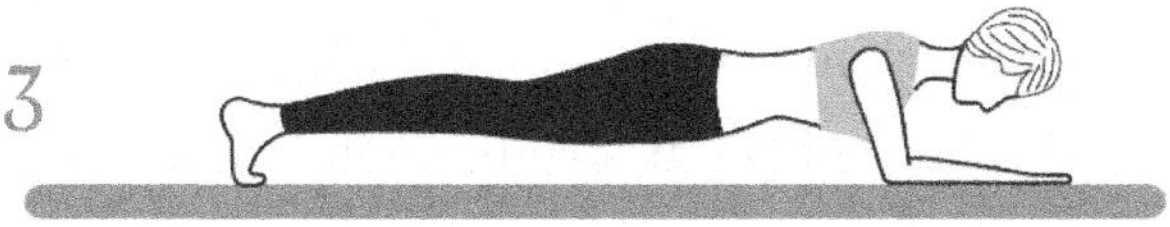

To tone your waist, use the same technique as above but do a lateral version:

1) Lie sideways to the ground, with your body weight on your right forearm and the edge of your right foot. Your glutes and abdominal muscles should be engaged.
2) When you have done 3 sets, repeat the exercise on the other side of your body (with your body weight on your left arm and left leg).

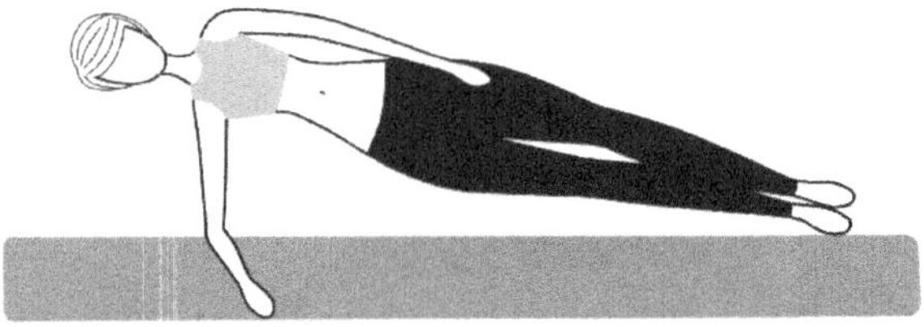

To strengthen your back muscles around your thorax and lumbar vertebrae, and to avoid pain due to bad daily posture:

1) Lie on the ground, with your legs hip width apart. Your knees should be bent at a right angle, your arms down by your side, your palms against the floor, and your chin clear.
2) Squeeze your glutes and lift your pelvis until your body is aligned with your thighs. All your body weight should be transferred to your head, shoulders, upper back, arms, and feet.

1

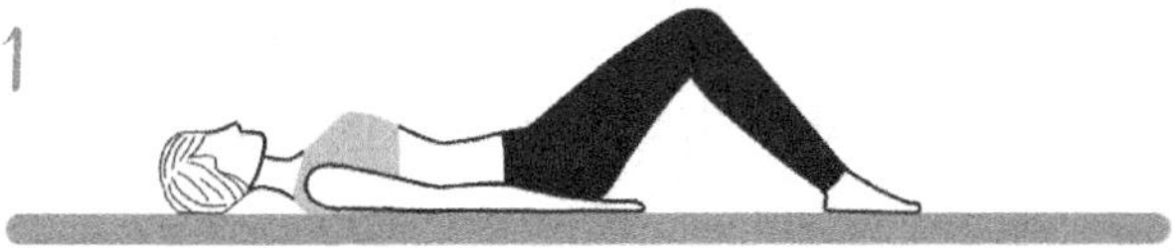

2

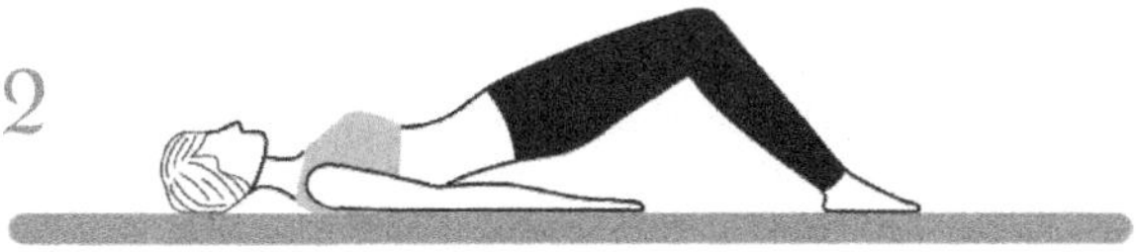

Note: For all the strengthening poses described here, it is important to remember to tilt your pelvis and flatten your back by trying to pull your pubis up toward your stomach and squeezing your glutes. This will protect your lower back. (If you are experienced, you can also try to contract your perineum during this exercise, to work "the" muscle that maintains the pelvic floor.)

Quantity: If you have a little pot belly you would like to get rid of, do strengthening exercises every day for 3 weeks (as well as reconsidering your diet, of course). For anyone else, incorporate these exercises into your workout. To begin with, do 3 sets of 30 seconds in a static position, with 30 seconds recovery time between each set. You can gradually increase the time you hold each pose until you reach 3 minutes.

Benefits: Goodbye little belly and hello hourglass waist! These strengthening exercises work the lower back and abdominals, acting on the postural muscles. They help to keep the pelvis well balanced and the spine stable.

- Chapter 17 -
Stretches

A good stretch helps you gain awareness of the different parts of the body that are being worked and lengthen any tight muscles. Despite common misconceptions, stretching also helps strengthen the muscles: look at the athletic bodies of yoga masters and teachers.

Stretch 1 – Opposite Arm and Leg Extension

1) Lie on the floor on your stomach with your legs and feet parallel, your arms extended out in front of you, your palms down to the ground, and your shoulders relaxed. Your abdominal muscles should be engaged. Inhale.
2) As you exhale, lift your right arm and left leg up from the ground. Extend them as if there are tethers pulling your right hand out in front of you and your left foot back behind you. *Make sure your pelvis stays flat on the floor and your legs parallel.*
3) As you inhale, come back to the starting position.
4) Repeat with your left arm and right leg.

Note: make sure your shoulders stay relaxed and your abdominal muscles engaged throughout this exercise. You shouldn't be arching your back, but lengthening it.

Quantity: Repeat 6 times.

Benefits: There's no better way to really relax your body than stretching out like a cat.

1

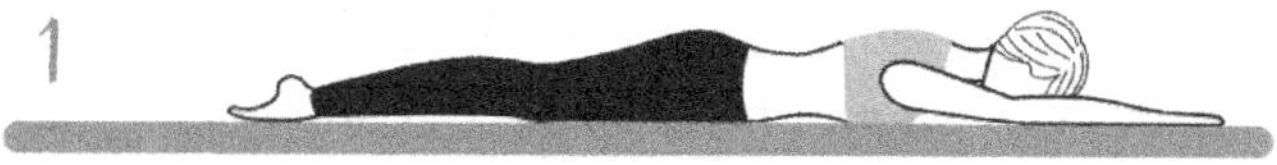

2

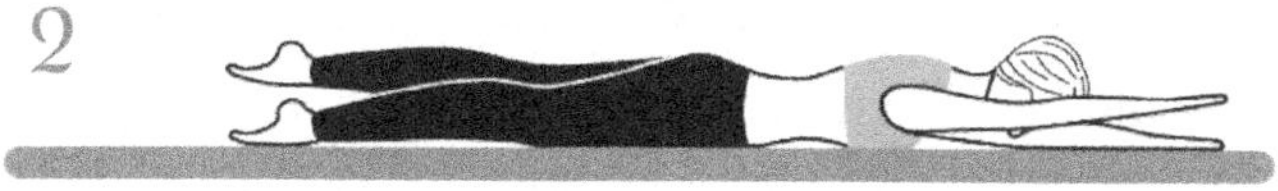

3

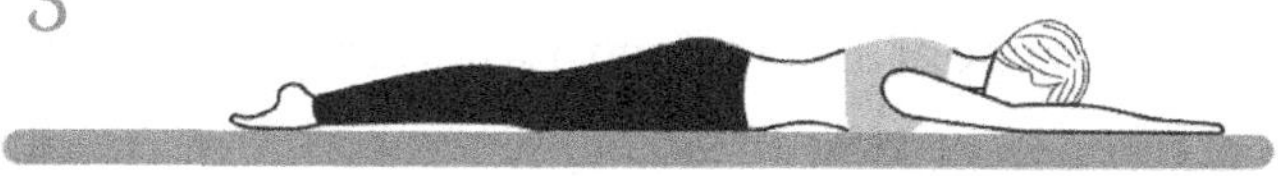

4

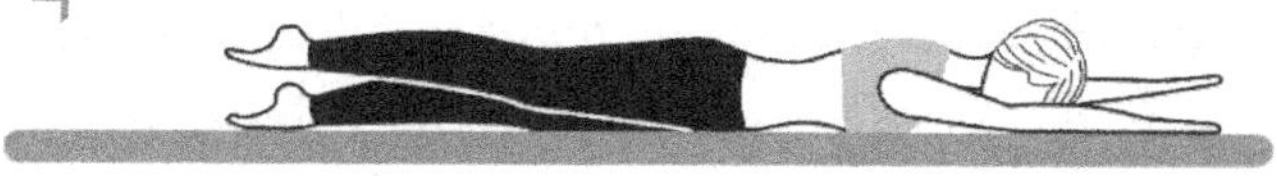

Stretch 2 - Sun Salutation (Yoga)

1) Begin by standing, looking straight ahead of you. Your upper body should be supple, your shoulders relaxed, your knees straight, and your feet hip width apart.
2) On an inhale, raise your arms above your head and imagine you are trying to reach the sky with your hands, keeping your chest broad and your shoulders down. Your palms should be facing each other, and your abdomen and glutes should be engaged. *Do 6 cycles of deep abdominal breathing, and with each inhale, try to stretch your hands up higher toward the sky, while opening your rib cage. Focus on your heart chakra (to find it, imagine a line between your nipples: your heart chakra is at the intersection of this line and your sternum).*
3) Interlace your fingers and turn your palms up toward the ceiling. On the next inhale, without shifting your pelvis or legs, lean your torso to the right, putting more weight on your right leg. Your left wrist should flex out as far as possible. Imagine you are creating more space between the ribs in your left ribcage and your spine is extending. *Note, from the side view, your body should still be on the same axis: the top of your body should not bend forward or backward.*
4) As you exhale, repeat the exercise, this time leaning to the left. *Gently repeat steps 3) and 4) over six breathing cycles.*

5) On the next exhale, return to position 2). Then, as you inhale, without shifting your pelvis or legs, swivel the top of your body backwards as though to bring your right shoulder over your butt. Remember to keep stretching your arms upward. As you exhale, pass through the neutral position and then repeat on your left side. *Repeat for 6 breathing cycles, then return to the starting position.*

Benefits: This sequence complements the Cat Pose (below) and helps to gently loosen up the spine.

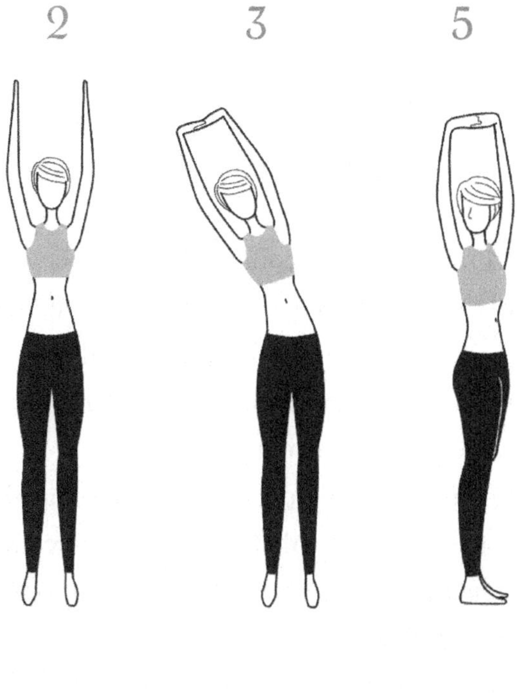

Stretch 3 - Cat Pose

Practiced as a stretch or warm-up during yoga, as well as in pilates, this exercise is directly inspired from the movement of cats. Think of the way a cat stretches its back when it wakes up. In humans, this stretch helps to loosen up the spine: try to stay aware of the movement of each vertebra and the space between them during the entire duration of this stretch.

1) Start on all fours. Your hands should be under your shoulders, your fingers pointing forward, and your arms straight. Your knees should be under your hips, with your legs slightly apart, and your feet pointing backward. Keep your spine straight, and your head and neck parallel to the ground.
2) As you inhale for 6 seconds, lift your coccyx and head up toward the ceiling, and dip your back as though your navel is being pulled down toward the ground. Your gaze should be turned upward. *Hold your breath for 6 seconds.*
3) Come back to the starting position.
4) Now exhale for 6 seconds, imagining that the middle of your back is being pulled up toward the ceiling. Let your neck relax and your head hang down. From a side view, you should be arching your back. *Hold your breath for 6 seconds.*

Make sure you keep your neck and shoulders relaxed during this exercise. If you have weak knees, you can put a (relatively thin) cushion or folded blanket under them.

Quantity: Repeat this "inhalation-exhalation" sequence 6 times.

Benefits: The cat sequence is beneficial for the neck and shoulders, as well as the dorsal muscles. The exercise is quite comprehensive, helping you to extend and flex your spine and is ideal when your back is tense from stress. Cat Pose is particularly useful for people who have round shoulders or who spend a lot of time in front of a computer screen.

1

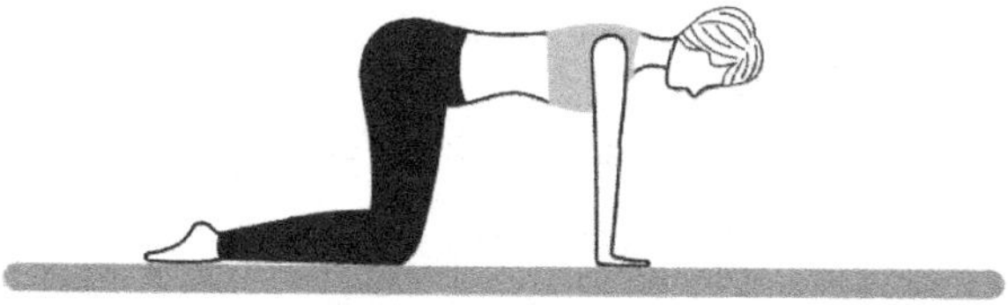

2

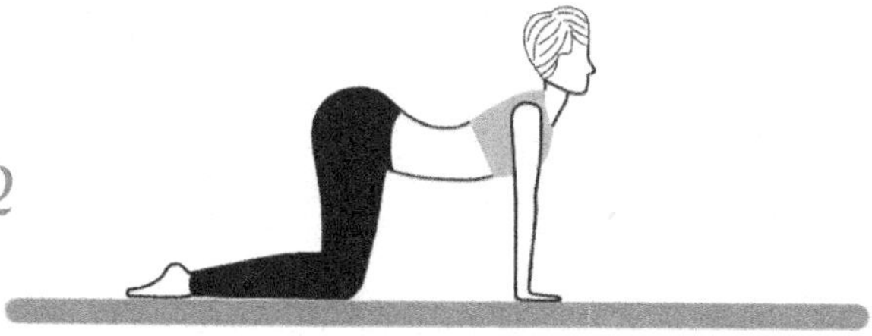

4

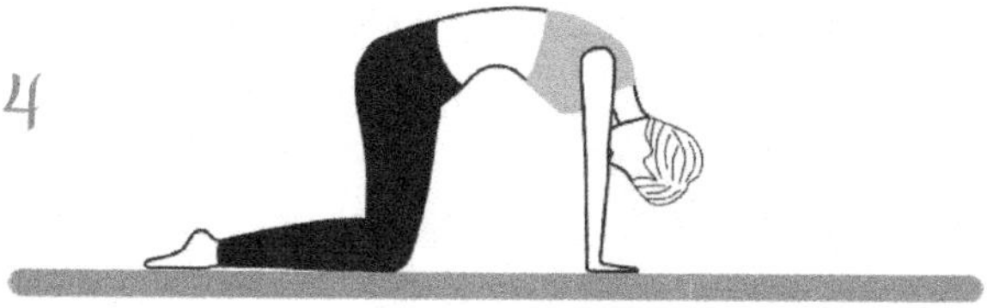

Stretch 4 - Knee to Chest

At the end of a long day, regardless of whether you have been wearing pumps or ballerina shoes, your lumbar spine may be tense and aching. If that is the case, this stretch is for you!

1) Lie on the ground with your head straight, your arms by your side, and your legs hip width apart.
2) Bend your legs, keeping your feet on the ground.
3) Gently bring your right knee up toward your head. Meanwhile, extend your left leg out on the ground.
4) As soon as you are able, catch your right leg and wrap your fingers around your knee. Then pull your right knee up as close as possible toward your chest. *Hold this position for 10 to 15 seconds.*
5) Now lower your arms back down beside your body and bring your legs back to position 2).
6) Repeat the sequence with your left leg.

Quantity: Work each leg 3 times.

Benefits: There is no better way to relieve lower back pain!

2

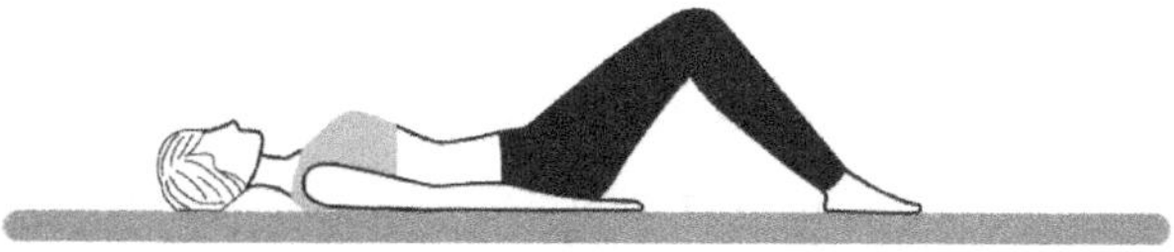

3 and 4

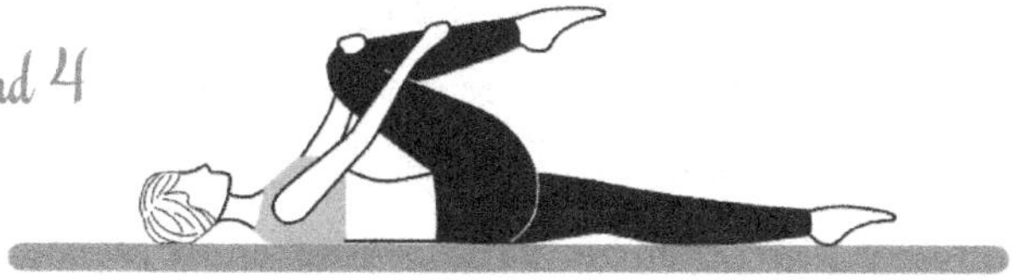

5

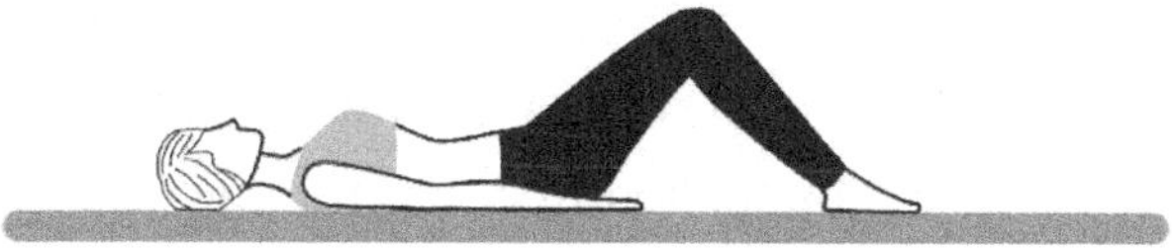

6

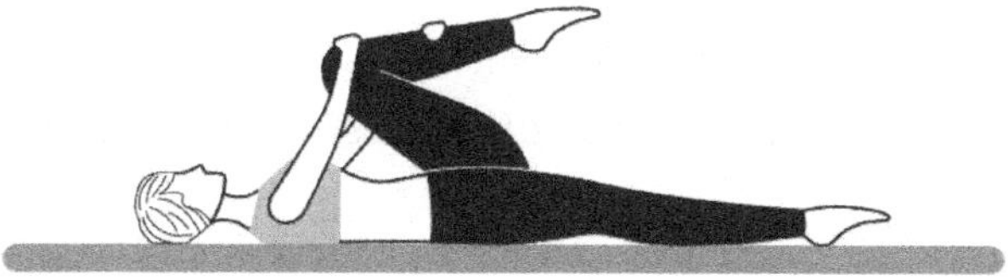

Stretch 5 - Ankle to Hand

1) Begin this exercise lying on your back, with your legs parallel and hip width apart, your knees bent, your arms outstretched with your palms down to the ground, and your shoulders relaxed.
2) Slowly turn your head to the right and lean your knees to the left until they touch the ground. Your shoulders should stay on the ground.
3) Holding this position, extend your right leg and lift it up until you are able to catch your right ankle in your left hand. *Hold the position for 30 seconds.*
4) Bend your right leg back down again.
5) Come back to the starting position, by bringing your knees and head back to the central position.
6) Repeat in the opposite direction, turning your head to the left and your knees to the right.

Note: While some exercises are not recommended if you have problems with your spine, this stretch should be particularly avoided if you suffer from back problems (especially damage to the vertebral discs).

Quantity: Repeat this stretch 3 times on each side.

Benefits: This exercise creates a lovely side stretch and gently massages the lower back.

1

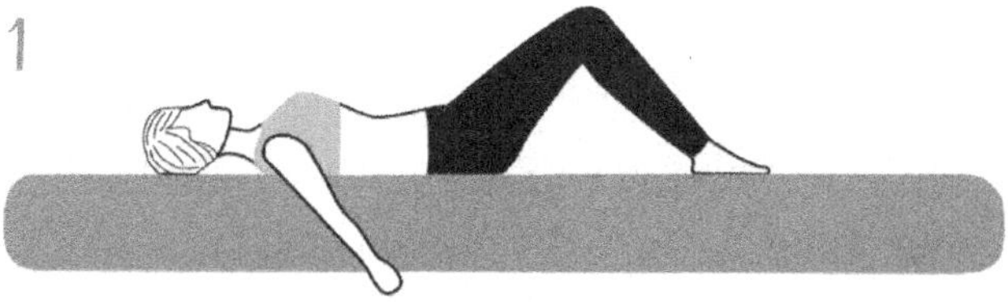

2

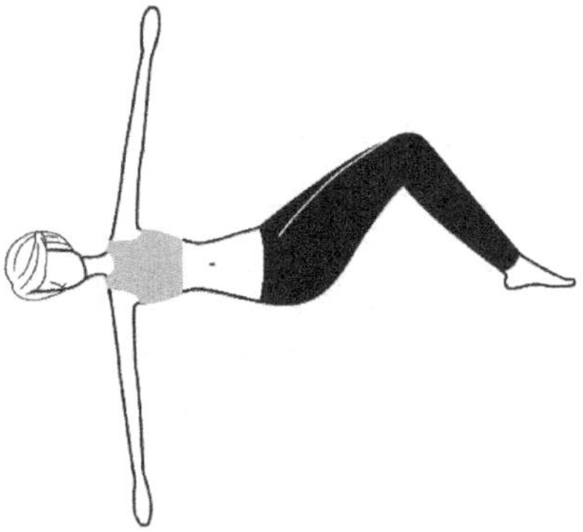

3

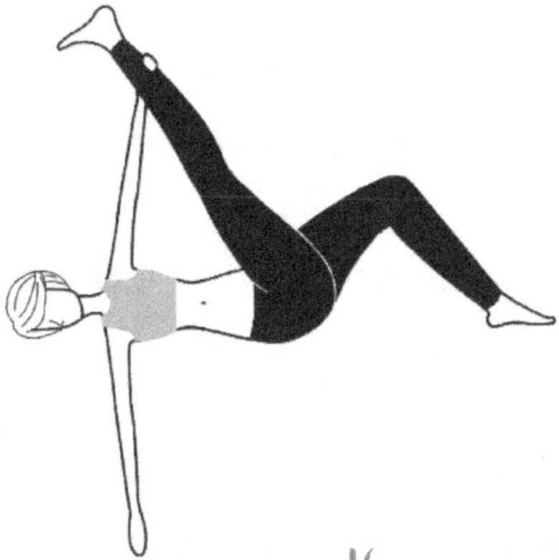

4

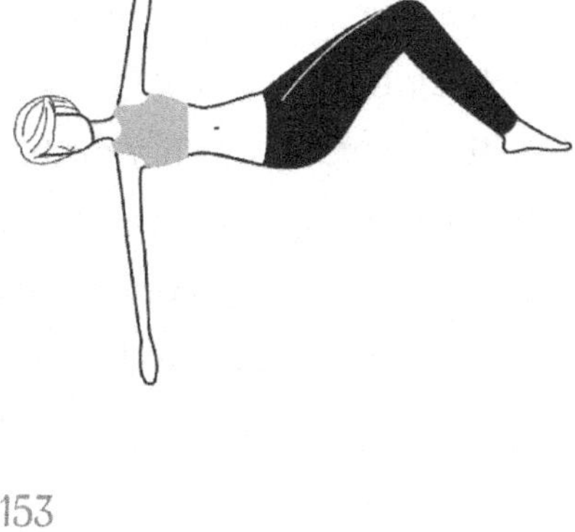

Stretch 6 – Revolved Abdomen Pose (Yoga)

1) Lie on your back, with your spine well extended. Slide your arms out to the sides so they are in line with your shoulders, turn your palms down to the ground, and keep your neck in a neutral position.
2) On an exhale, bend your legs up, keeping them together, and lift your thighs as close as possible to your stomach. *Hold for 2 breaths.*
3) On the next exhale, gently sweep your legs to the left, and turn your head to the right. Then on the inhale, bring your legs and head back to position 2). On the following exhale, sweep your legs to the right, and turn your head to the left. Return to position 2). *Breathing deeply, do 6 right-left sequences. Be careful not to lift your shoulders off the floor.*
4) Holding the same position, stretch your legs out on the floor, keeping them together.
5) Now as you exhale, sweep your legs (still outstretched) to the left and turn your head to the right. *Hold the position for 6 breaths.* Then as you inhale, bring your legs and head back to the center. On the next exhale, sweep your legs to the right, and turn your head to the left. *Hold the position for 6 breaths.* Come back to the center. *Note, once again, that you should not lift your shoulders from the ground.*
6) Return to the neutral position, lying on the ground.

Benefits: As with all bending exercises, this stretch massages the organs by compression. The twisting movement also helps relieve any stiffness in the lower back.

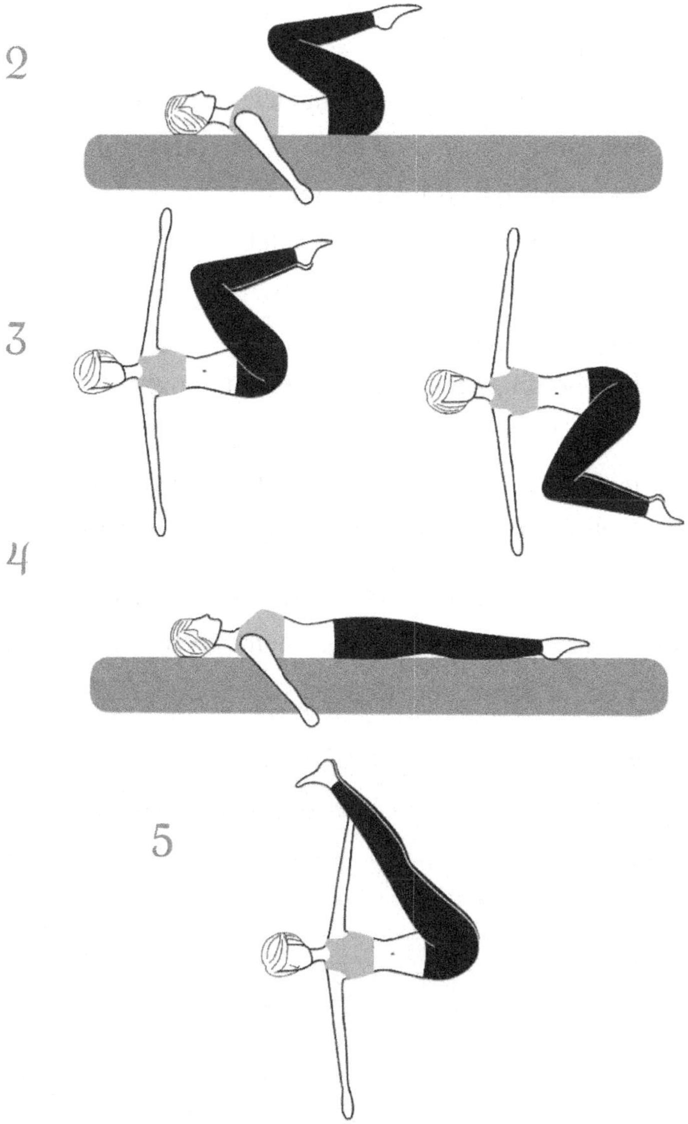

Stretch 7 - The Lying Half Lotus

This exercise is beneficial if you suffer from a stiff lower back.

1) Lie on your back with your arms down beside your body (palms to the ground), your legs hip width apart, and your knees bent.
2) Lift your right leg and rotate it at the hip so your right ankle rests just above your left knee. (Your right hip should be open, in a half-lotus position.)
3) Lift your torso until your hands can catch your left thigh just above the knee (at the distal hamstring muscle attachment).
4) Still holding your left thigh, lower your head and torso back down to the ground. Now bring your left leg as far as possible toward your chest to stretch out the muscles of your right buttock. *Hold the position for 30 seconds.*

During this stretch, make sure the lower leg (the one that is in the starting position) stays in alignment with the corresponding shoulder on the same side of your body.

A variant exists to stretch the glutes, the lumbar spine, and the hamstrings: the lower leg remains outstretched and in alignment with the body.

Quantity: Repeat 3 times on each side.

Benefits: This stretch helps relieve any tension in the lower back and stretches the glutes.

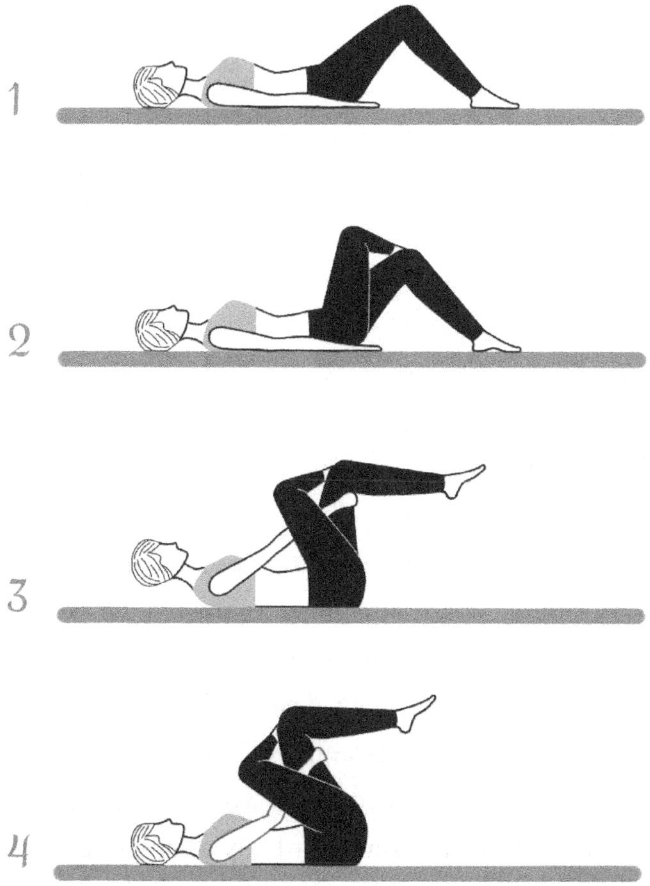

Stretch 8 - The Butterfly

The butterfly is a stretch practiced by dancers, in the same way as the splits. This pose helps avoid the aches and stiffness of the hips that are often felt after a ballet class or after wearing high heels for a prolonged period. Variant B also helps stretch the spine.

1) Sit down on the floor. Place the soles of your feet together. The lateral (external) edges of your feet should be against the ground, and your heels should be about 12 inches from your pubis.
2) Sit up straight and breathe in deeply. *Don't press on your knees to lower them! The more relaxed you are, the closer your knees will come to the floor.*
3) Variant A: If you are comfortable in this pose and your knees touch the ground, you can try bringing your heels closer to your pubis.
4) Variant B: staying in Butterfly Pose, imagine your spine is very straight and is stretching up toward the sky as though you are creating space between each vertebra. Lift your arms up above your head. Then, holding this position, lean forward over your legs until you are lying down flat. Keep your arms outstretched, as if your fingers are trying to move as far away from your body as possible, but without stiffening your shoulders. Breathe deeply and relax.
5) If you are really flexible, you can even combine variants A and B.

Quantity: Hold this pose for 3 or 4 minutes when you feel the need to stretch

Benefits: The aim of this exercise is to loosen up the hips and to stretch out the spine (depending on which variant you do).

1 and 2

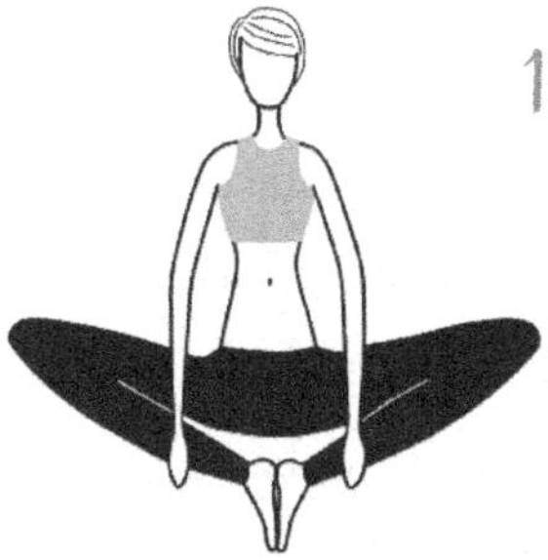

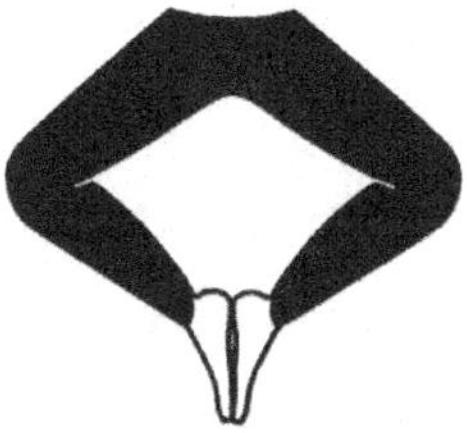

Variant A

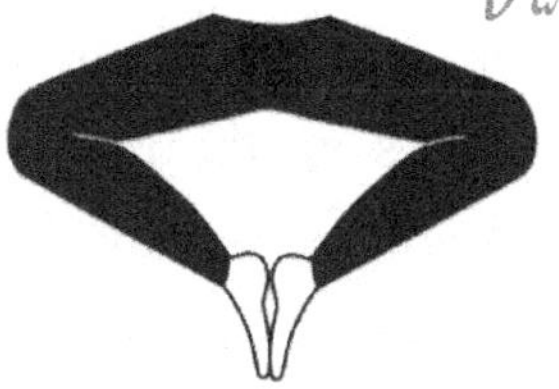

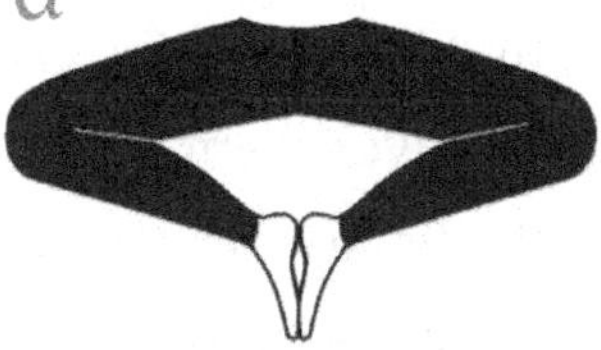

Variant B

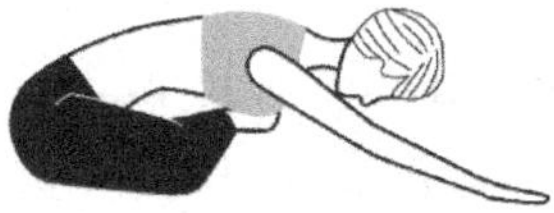

Stretch 9 - Cobbler's Pose (Yoga)

The previous dance stretch is derived from this yoga pose. If you can do the butterfly and its variants easily, then try Cobbler's Pose!

1) Sit on the floor with your legs outstretched together in front of you and your toes pointing toward you. Your arms should be down by your side, your torso perpendicular to the floor, your shoulders relaxed, and your chin clear. Feel the contact with the ground at the back of your knees.
2) Rotate your legs outward and bend your knees (so they are pointing outward). Now bring your heels up toward your pubis, pulling the soles of your feet together. Feel your spine stretch. To bring your knees closer to the ground, relax and try to lower them as you exhale.
3) Interlace your fingers and wrap them over your toes, as if to cover them. Place your elbows on the inside of your thighs and lean forward, until your forehead touches the floor. *Hold the pose for 6 breaths, then straighten up slowly.*

Benefits: This pose works stiff hips and the spine, just like the Butterfly Pose in dance. But Cobbler's Pose allows you to work the hips and adductor muscles in the thighs more deeply. This pose also helps improve the circulation of energy in the pelvis by massaging the organs.

2

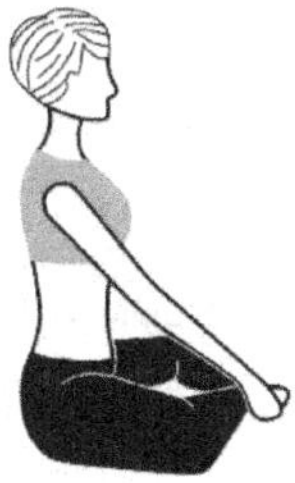

3

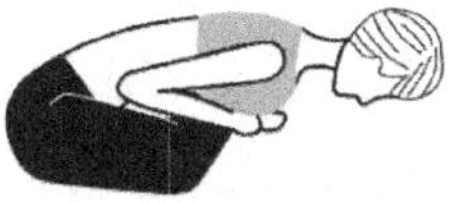

Stretch 10 - Standing Forward Bend (Yoga)

1) Standing in Mountain Pose, inhale as you lift your arms out wide and raise them up above your head, pressing the palms together.
2) Keeping your legs soft, lean forward, folding only at the hips until your head comes into contact with your knees. If possible, straighten your knees. Lay your hands on either side of your feet. Your neck and upper body should be relaxed. *Do 6 deep breathing cycles, visualizing your spine lengthening.*
3) Bend your knees slightly to gently lift your body back up again, keeping your spine fully extended.

Benefits: This pose helps work the pelvis and stretch out the back of the legs and lower spine. Holding your head down for a few breaths brings a "fresh" blood supply to your head, improving circulation in the brain and eyes.

1

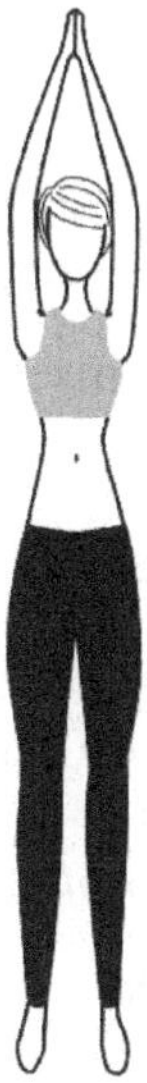

2

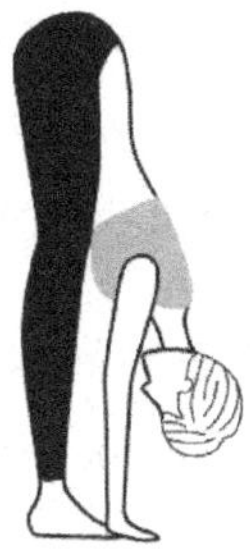

Stretch 11 – Grand Plié in Second Position

1) Stand with your hands on your hips, your shoulders relaxed, and your feet about 20 inches apart (some people may be able to go further).
2) Rotate your legs at your hips so your feet are pointing to the sides. (If you are very supple, your feet will be in alignment with your shoulders.) Your legs should be firm and straight.
3) Engage your abdominals and glutes and bend your knees until they are over your toes. Exhale.
4) Straighten your knees (and go back up) on the next inhale.

Note: the knees tend to drop forward, so make sure they stay in alignment with the tibia and femur as you bend and straighten.

Quantity: Repeat 6 times.

Benefits: This exercise helps to stretch the hips, glutes, and thighs.

1

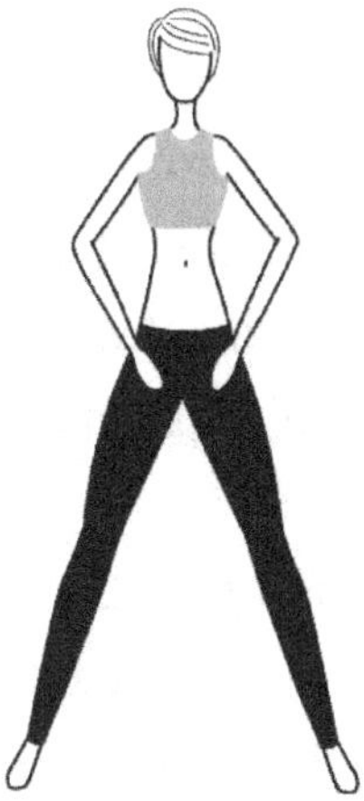

2

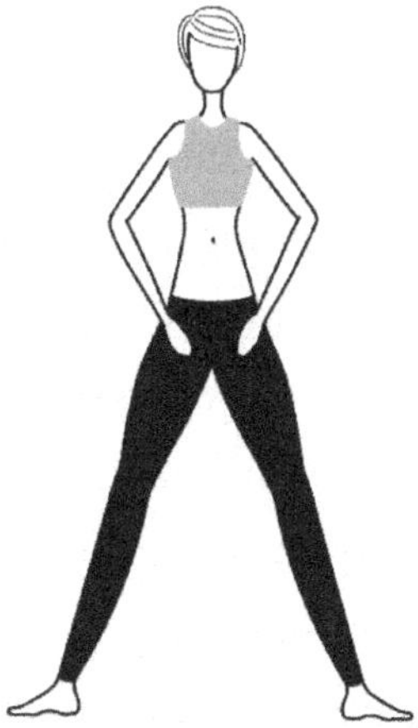

3

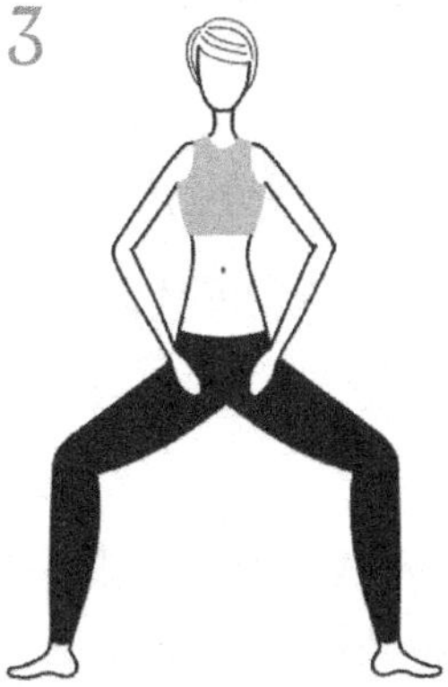

4

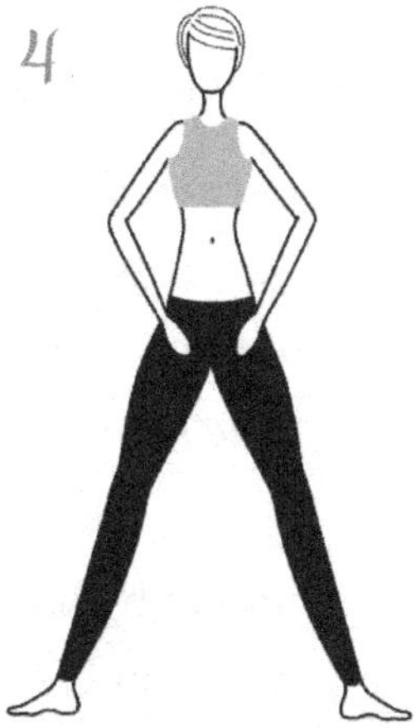

Stretch 12 – The Frog

This stretch isn't for everybody, but it allows you to work the hips well!

1) Start on the ground on all fours: your arms should be firm and straight, your hands positioned under your shoulders, your spine straight, your head in alignment with your body, your knees positioned under your hips, and your feet parallel.
2) Slowly slide your knees out on the ground, keeping your toes together. Your hips should form a 90° angle, and your pelvis should be as close to the ground as possible. Hold the position for a moment.
3) Return to the starting position 1), lifting your pelvis as you gently bring your knees back under your hips.

Note: your pelvis should be as close as possible to the ground, your spine as straight as possible, and your head in alignment. If you don't lower your pelvis enough toward the ground, you could arch your back too much and injure it.

Quantity: Begin by holding the position for 10 seconds, then work progressively up to 20 seconds.

Benefits: Like the Butterfly, the Frog is the ideal pose for stretching the hips and encouraging them to open.

1

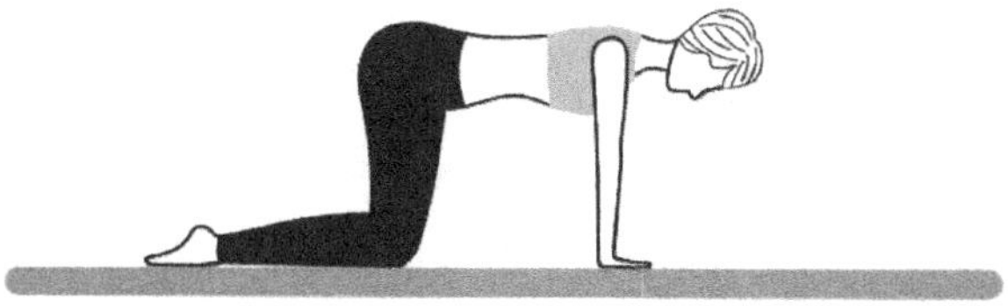

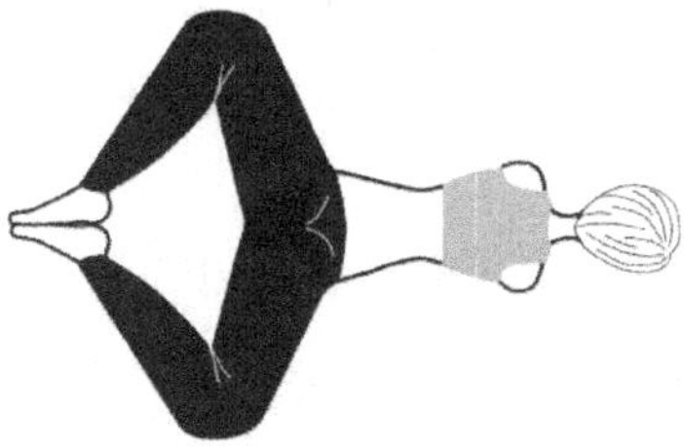

2

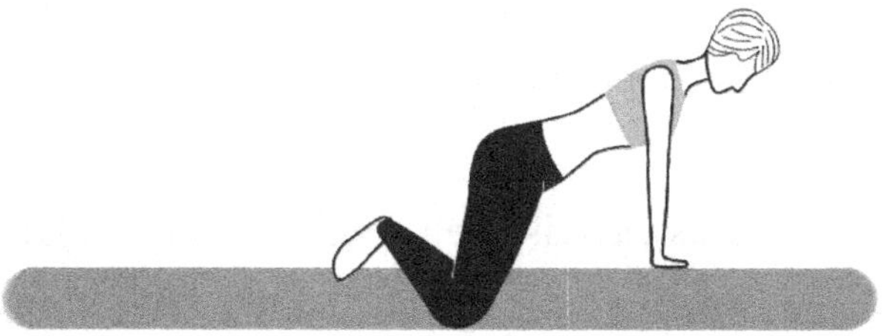

Stretch 13 – Cross-Legged Forward Fold (Yoga)

1) Sit on the floor with your legs crossed, your right leg in front of your left leg. Try to make sure that each of your feet is level with the knee of your opposite leg, and that your knees are not higher than your hips. If necessary, place folded blankets under your butt so your hip joints are at the right height.
2) Your spine should be straight and your neck clear. Place your hands palm down on your knees. *Do 3 cycles of deep breathing.*
3) Put your hands on the ground in front of you.
4) Slide your hands forward until your forearms touch the ground. Rest your forehead on the ground. *Do 6 breathing cycles.*
5) Slowly pull back up again, letting your hands slide back along the ground. Repeat the exercise with your legs crossed the opposite way.

Benefits: This exercise helps soften the hips and the inner thighs. It is an ideal position for meditation, allowing you to focus on your breathing.

2

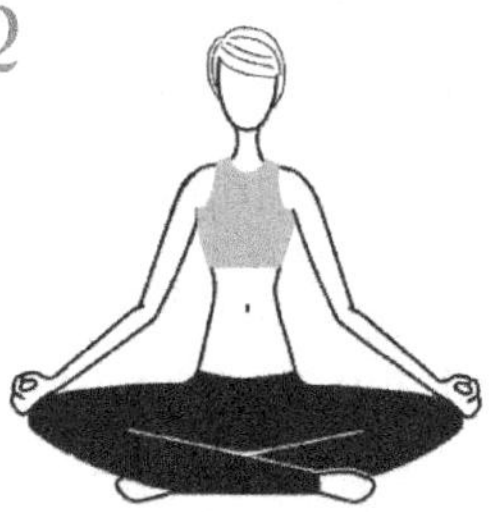

3

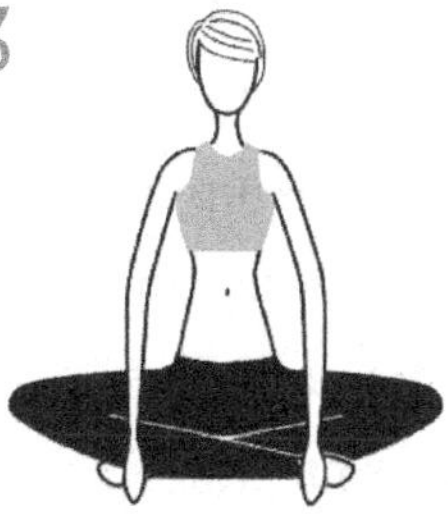

4

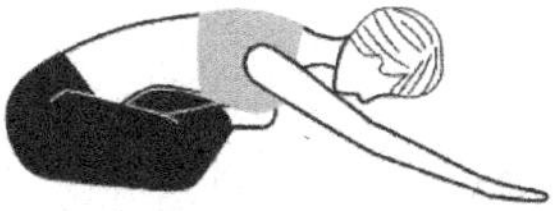

Stretch 14 - Crescent Moon Pose (Yoga)

1) Start kneeling up, with your legs together, your arms down by your side, and your abdominal muscles engaged.
2) Step your right foot forward so your thigh is parallel to the ground. Place your hands on your right knee. Shift your body weight onto your right leg as you move forward, keeping your torso straight. Can you feel the stretch in your left thigh? (If you are very flexible, move your right leg further forward.)
3) As though drawing a circle, stretch your arms out wide and raise them above your head so the palms come together. Then stretch your arms up as far as possible, tilting them slightly backward, as though your fingers are trying to reach the sky, while your chest opens and broadens. Direct your gaze up to your forefingers. Don't put too much pressure on your shoulders and try to keep your pelvis as low as possible to the ground. *Do 6 cycles of breathing.*
4) Return to position 1) on the next exhale, then repeat the exercise with your left leg in front of you.

Benefits: This pose stretches the pelvis and iliopsoas muscles, as well as the front of the thighs. The little bonus? It revitalizes the kidneys and liver.

1

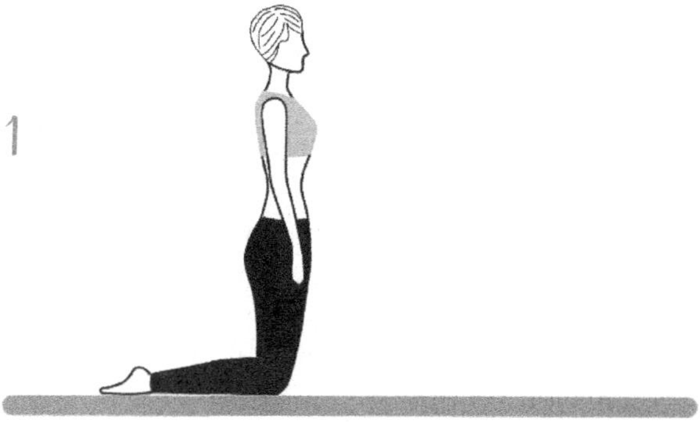

2

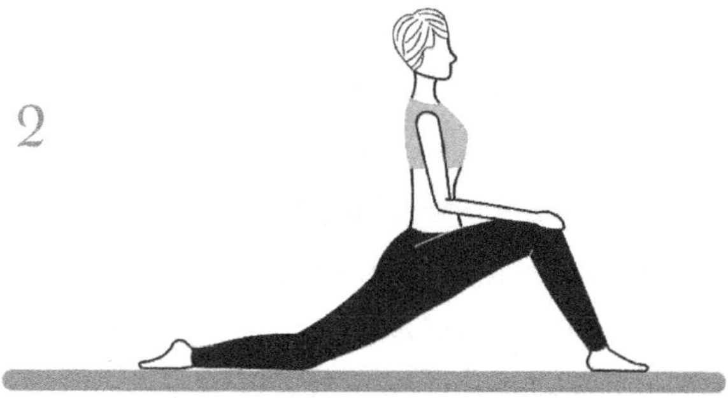

3

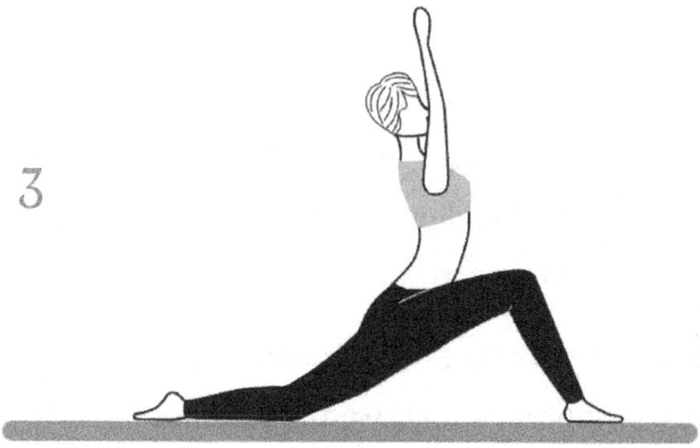

Stretch 15 - Chest to Thigh

An ideal exercise if you want to improve your flexibility…

1) Begin by sitting on the ground, with your legs stretched out together in front of you. Your spine should be straight and perpendicular to the ground, your head straight, your chin clear, and your hands on your thighs.
2) Very gently, keeping your spine lengthened, lower your chest down as close as you can to your thighs. As you are lowering yourself down, extend your spine as if you have a string attached to the top of your head. Your head must stay in alignment: your chin should be neither tucked under nor lifted. Your hands can slide forward along your legs. *If you are struggling, imagine you stay in starting position 1), and that the only movement is a forward rotation from your hips.*
3) When you can't go down any lower keeping your spine straight, and only then, bend the top of your spine and head down over your legs. You can let your hands rest on your shins, beside your legs, or if you are very flexible, under the soles of your feet.

Instead of leaving your feet as they are, you can also do the same exercise pulling your toes up toward your knees.

Note: don't cheat! Make sure you keep your legs completely straight throughout the exercise, and don't bend or tense your upper body! And as a reminder: the more you force, the less far you will be able to lean down over your legs. The more relaxed you are, the more deeply you will breathe, and the further you will be able to take the stretch.

Quantity: Hold the position for 30 seconds to start with, increasing up to 1 or 2 minutes if you are able to.

Benefits: This exercise is quite comprehensive and helps stretch and loosen up the spine, the hip joints, the glutes, the back of the legs, the knees, and the thighs. Ideal after a day perched on a pair of 4 inch heels...

1

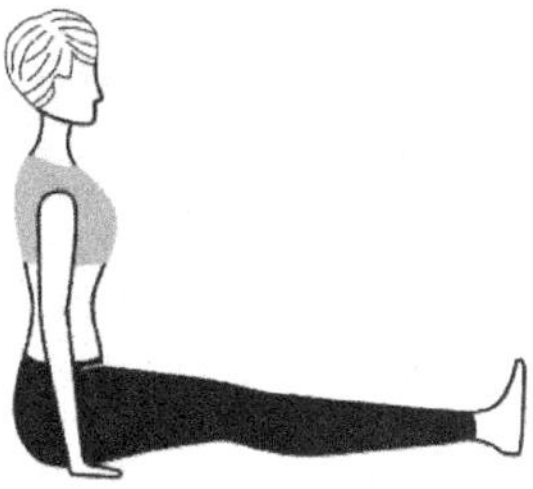

2

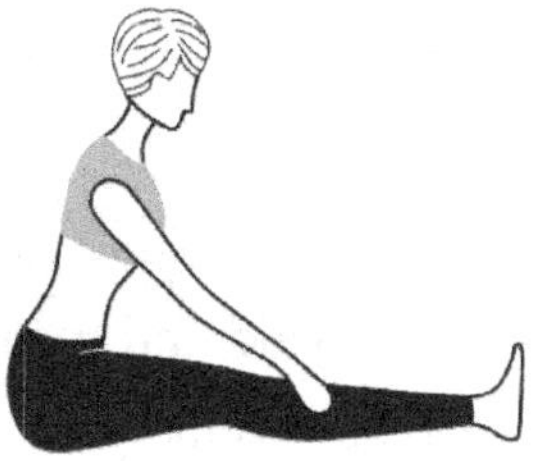

3

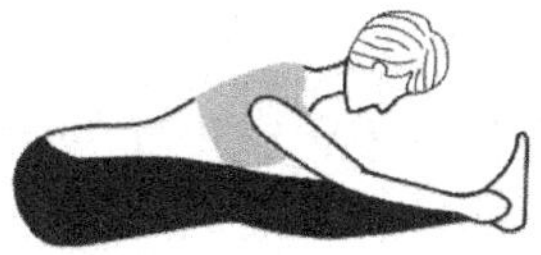

Stretch 16 - Chest over Crossed Thighs

1) The starting position is identical to that in the previous stretch: your legs should be parallel, your back and head straight, your arms by your side, and your palms down to the ground.
2) Put your hands under your right knee to lift it and place your right leg over your left leg. (Your two legs should touch at the thighs.)
3) Slide your hands down to your right ankle and bend your body forward at the hips, being careful to keep your spine as straight as possible. Your neck should stay in alignment with your spine.
4) When you can't bring your abdomen any closer to your thighs, and only then, bend the upper part of your chest and head over your right leg.
5) Gently return to the starting position, beginning by raising your head and then your chest, as you lower your right leg to the ground.
6) Repeat with the left leg.

Note: your legs should be straight, but be careful not to hyperextend your knees or over contract your quadriceps.

Quantity: Hold each intermediate position for 5 seconds, and the final position for 10 seconds. Don't repeat the exercise: one sequence per leg is enough.

Benefits: This exercise allows you to effectively work the hips, glutes, and inner thighs, but it is especially beneficial for the calves: when you wear high heels often, the calf muscles tend to contract and shorten. This exercise helps stretch them.

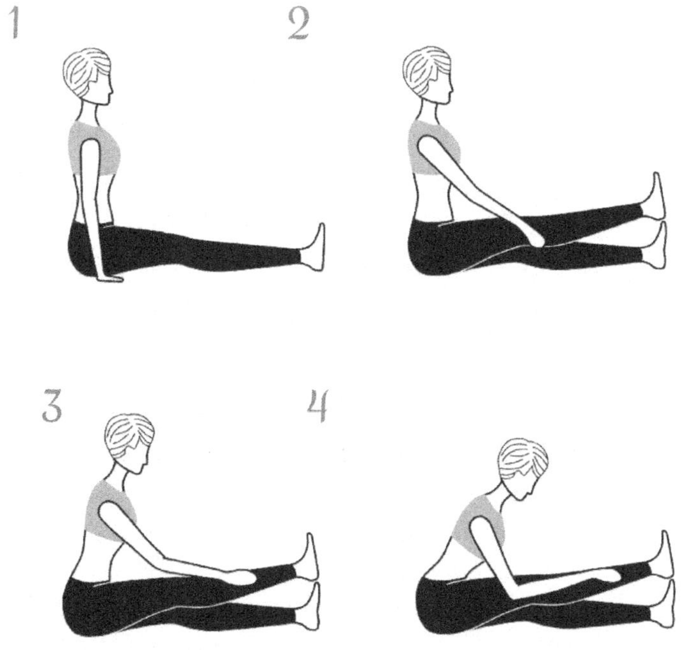

Stretch 17 - Downward Dog (Yoga)

1) Starting in Mountain Pose, raise your arms above your head as you inhale.
2) On the exhale, lean forward, hinging only at the hips, until your hands are flat down on either side of your feet and your head is at your knees. Your fingers should be pointing forward.
3) On the next exhale, step one foot back and then the other, until there is a 30 to 35 inch gap between your hands and feet. Gently lift your pelvis. Your sit bones should be pointing toward the ceiling, your arms and legs straight and firm, your chin tucked under, your neck lengthened, and your shoulder blades turned outward. If you are flexible and the soles of your feet touch the ground easily, then step your feet back further. *Do 3 cycles of 6 breaths.*
4) On an inhale, step your feet forward to help you straighten back up again.

Benefits: This well-known Downward Dog pose helps bring oxygen to the head, and stretches the spine, the muscles at the back of the thighs, the back of the knees, and the shoulders.

1

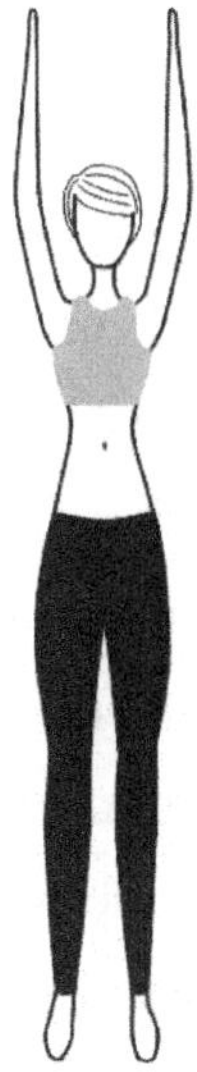

2

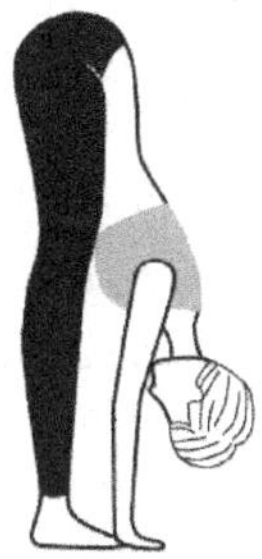

3

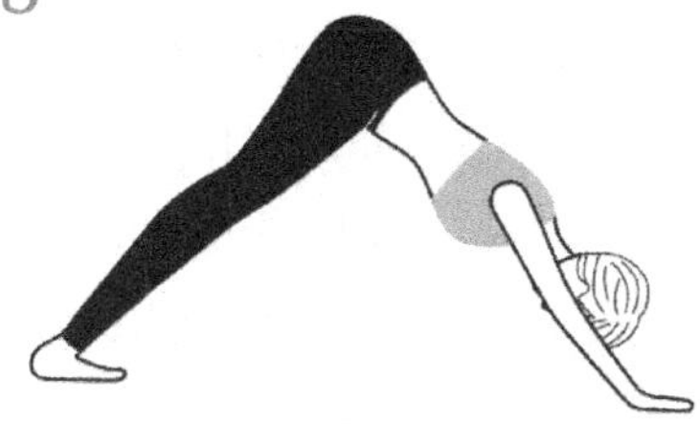

Stretch 18 – Extended Hand-to-Big-Toe Pose (Yoga)

1) Starting in Mountain Pose, transfer your body weight onto your left leg. Place your left hand on your hip. Lift your right leg, bending your knee until you can catch your big toe with three fingers of your right hand (thumb, forefinger, and middle finger). Without lifting your right hip, extend your right leg out in front of you. *Focusing on a point in the distance, do 6 cycles of deep breathing.*
2) Rotate your right leg around to the side, again without lifting your hip. Turn your head and eyes to the left. *Hold for 6 breathing cycles.*
3) Bring your leg back in front of you. Release your leg and put your right hand on your hip. Try not to let your leg fall heavily. Use your abdominal muscles to retain it. Point your foot and raise your leg as high as possible, keeping it straight. Try to stay stable, without leaning backwards. Imagine a string from the top of your head pulling it up toward the ceiling. *Hold for 3 breathing cycles.*
4) Set your foot back down and repeat on the other side.

Benefits: While this exercise is practiced in yoga classes, it is also often used in classical dance to stretch the pelvis, improve balance, and increase the flexibility of the hips and the inside and back of the thighs. By keeping your leg stretched out in front of you without holding it, you work your leg muscles and abdominals.

1

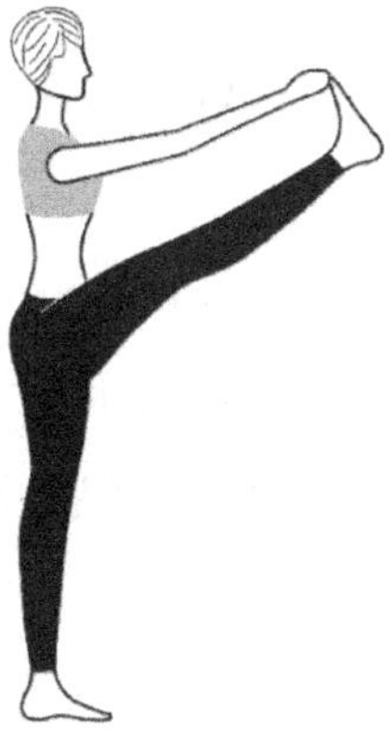

2

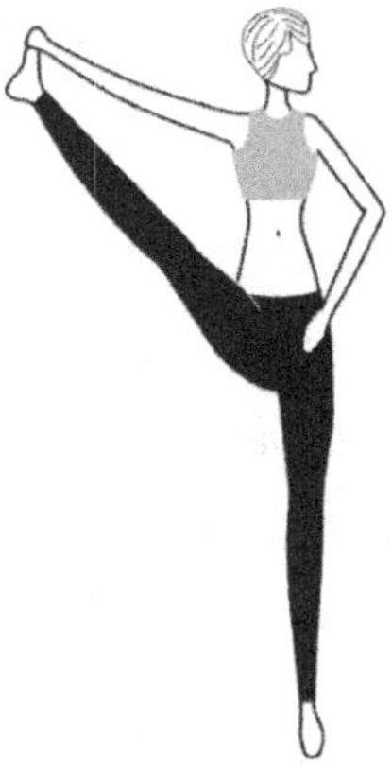

3

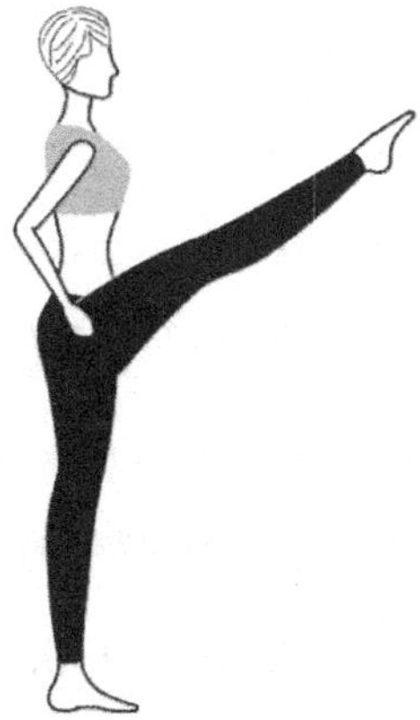

Stretch 19 - The Perfect Pose (Yoga)

Sit down on the floor with your legs stretched out together in front of you, your toes pointing toward you, your arms by your side, your torso perpendicular to the floor, your shoulders relaxed, and your chin clear.

Bend your right leg to bring it up to your left thigh: your right heel should be lying against your pubis. Bend your left leg and bring your left heel up against your right ankle. Point your right foot. Place your hands on your knees, and put your thumb and index finger together.

Breathe deeply and feel your spine stretch: your pelvis should be firmly down on the ground, while the top of your head stretches up toward the ceiling. Keep your shoulders relaxed. In order to stretch the vertebrae of your spine, you can bend your head forward slightly.

Variant: your left leg bends and passes over your right leg. Your left foot then rests in the space between your right thigh and calf.

Be careful not to let your pelvis roll forward: remember to lengthen your spine and keep your abdominal muscles engaged.

Try to switch your legs around each time you do this pose.

Quantity: In a standard session, you do several breathing cycles before moving on to a new pose. But if you would like to do fifteen minutes' meditation, you can hold this pose.

Benefits: Of course this pose helps soften the hips, knees, and ankles. You can also feel the increased blood supply to your lower spine and genitals.

1

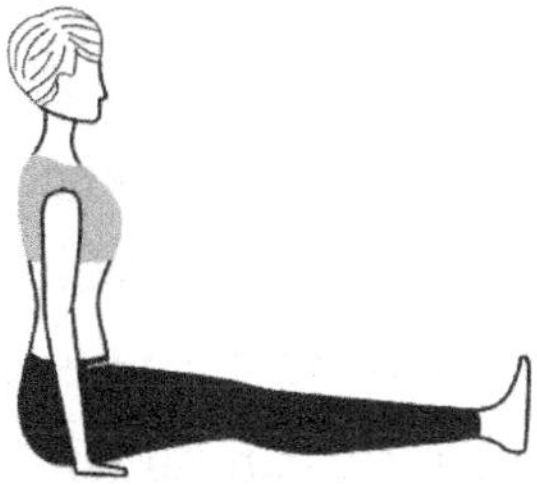

2 and 3

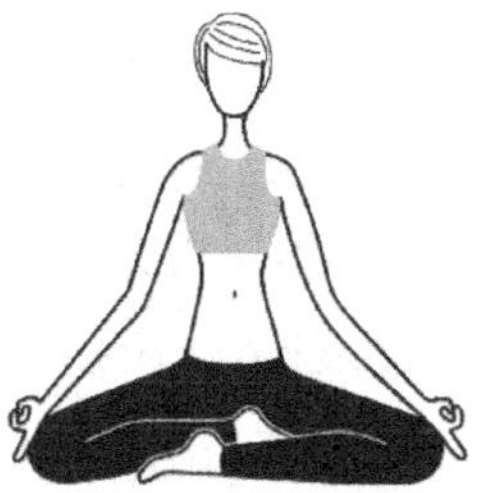

Stretch 20 - Single-Leg-Folded Seated Forward Fold (Yoga)

1) Sit on the floor with your legs stretched out together in front of you, your toes pointing toward you, your arms by your side, your torso perpendicular to the floor, your shoulders relaxed, and your chin clear. Feel the contact of the back of your knees on the ground.
2) Bend your right knee and bring your right foot up toward your hip. With your right hand, push your calf outwards. Your thighs should be parallel, and your knees close to each other. Your right foot should be pointing inward, with the back of your foot against the floor. Try to point the toes of your left foot up toward you. Be careful not to lift your butt from the floor: you should be able to feel your sit bones on the ground and your two iliac bones should be level. *Caution: if you ever feel pain in your right ankle, stop and change position.*
3) On the exhale, lean forward by extending your spine, until your forehead rests on your left shin. Your shoulders should be relaxed, and your back broad (push your shoulder blades outward). *Hold the pose for 6 breaths.*
4) On the inhale, straighten slowly up and return to the starting position. Repeat the sequence with your left leg.

Caution, you could injure your knee if the foot of your bent leg is pointing outward.

Benefits: A pose that loosens up the hips, knees and ankles, making it ideal for people with sciatica. As with all the bending poses (forward folds), it helps to massage the organs.

1

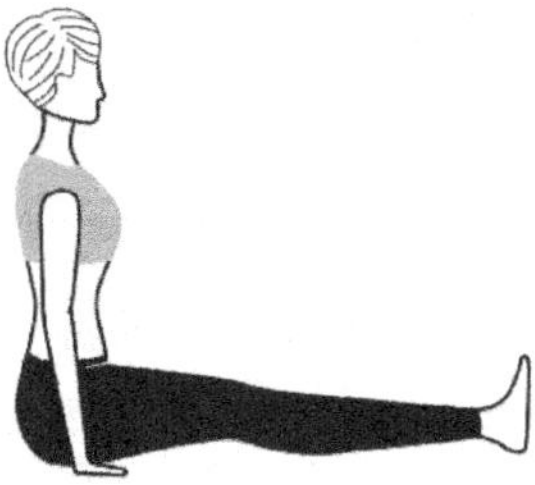

2

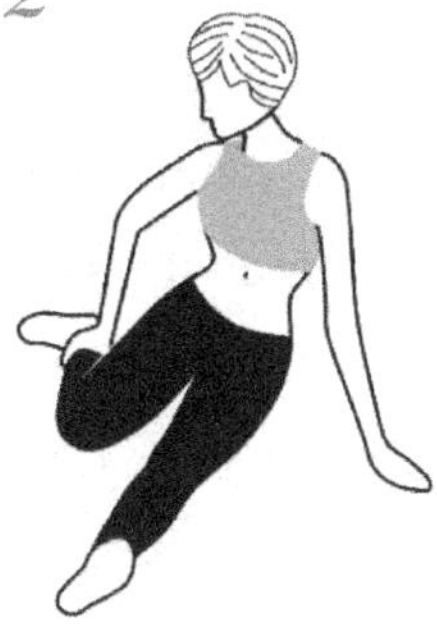

3

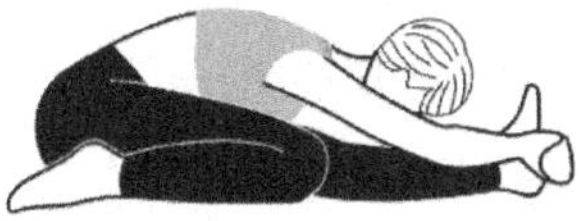

Stretch 21 - Head-to-Knee with Stretched Toes Pose (Yoga)

1) Sit down on the floor, with your legs stretched out together in front of you, your toes pointing toward you, your arms by your side, your torso perpendicular to the floor, your shoulders relaxed, and your chin clear. Feel the contact with the ground at the back of your knees.
2) Rotate your right leg outward and bend your knee. Bring your toes up to your pubis with your right hand (your arm should pass between your thigh and your calf). (The lateral edge of your foot should be against your pubis, while your toes touch the ground.) Now lift your heel up over your toes with your left hand (imagine you are pushing your heel forward). The toes of your left foot should be pointing toward you. Sit up, so that your spine is straight and lengthened. *If you are not flexible, hold this position for 6 breathing cycles. You can always try to go further in another session: flexibility improves with practice. For the more flexible, let's continue...*
3) As you exhale, lean forward, extending your left arm and shoulder, so your right hand can catch hold of the bottom of your left foot. Rest your head on your left shin. Feel your spine lengthen as if the top of your head is being pulled toward your left foot. Use your left hand to catch hold of your right wrist under your left foot. Lift your gaze to the toes of your left foot. *Hold the position for 6 breaths.*

4) On an inhale, return to position 1), then repeat on the other side.

There is a variant to this pose for an advanced level of difficulty: in position 3, you can rest your chin on your shin and look up toward your toes

Benefits: This is a comprehensive pose that stretches the toes, the Achilles tendons, the knees, the muscles at the back of the thighs, and the hips. Because it is a bending pose, it massages and tones the organs.

1

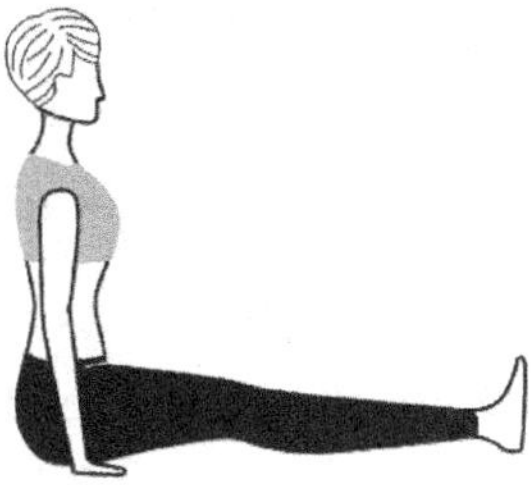

2

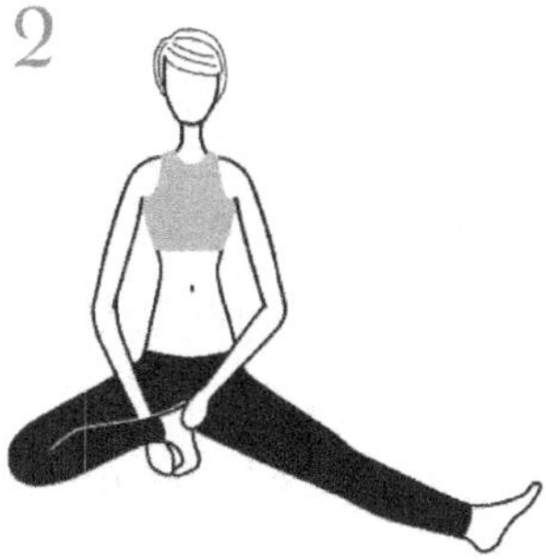

3

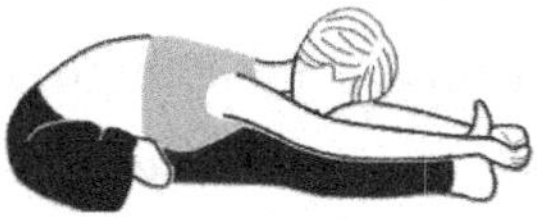

Stretch 22 - Inverted Splits

This exercise is practiced with one bent leg resting on the ground to help protect the lumbar spine by preventing your back from arching. The idea of the exercise is to bring your leg as close as possible toward you with each bend and extension.

1) Lie on the floor, with your arms down by your side, your legs hip width apart, and your head in alignment with your spine. Bend your legs so your knees form a right angle.
2) Extend your right leg and lift it up toward your chest until you can catch hold of it. To make sure you have a good hold, place your hands near your knees, one under your thigh, and the other under the top of your calf.
3) To catch hold of your leg you will probably have sat up a little, so now while still holding your leg, lie down, relax, and make sure your pelvis is firmly down on the ground. We often try to use our shoulders to help us: be careful not to do this here and to keep your shoulders relaxed. *Hold this position for 30 seconds.*
4) Bend your right knee and pull your thigh up as close as possible to your chest.
5) Then, trying to move your thigh as little as possible (and therefore your femur), extend your leg. *Hold for 30 seconds.*

Note: don't forget that with stretches, the more you relax, the further you can take the stretch.

If you are not very flexible and you aren't able to extend your leg while holding it, you can wrap a towel behind your calf. This will help you pull your leg closer to your chest while keeping it extended, without tensing your back or neck.

Quantity: 6 sets of "bends and extensions" for each leg

Benefits: This exercise allows you to completely stretch out the entire back of the leg (hamstrings) as far as the glutes.

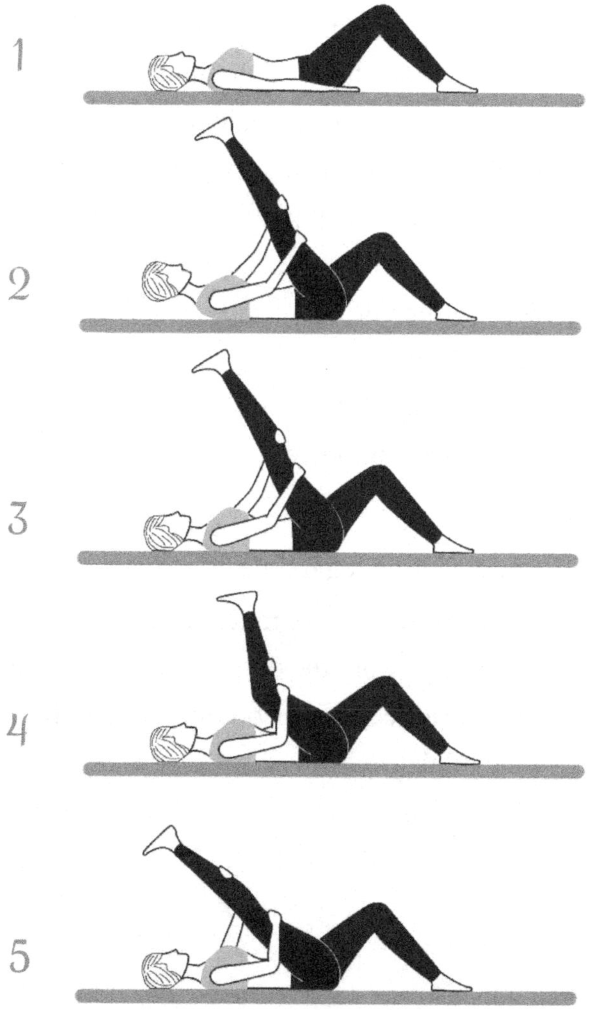

Stretch 23 - Lunge

This stretch particularly targets the muscles at the front of the thighs.

1) Begin by standing with your feet parallel and hip width apart, your arms down by your side, and your head straight.
2) Take a big step forward with your right leg. Both your legs should be bent. But be careful: your front knee must stay at a 90° angle. This helps protect your knee.
3) Keep your arms outstretched at shoulder height on either side of your body to help maintain your balance. Your spine should be straight and as perpendicular to the ground possible, while your back knee is as close to the ground as possible.
4) Hold the position for about ten seconds, then repeat the same exercise with your left leg in front.
5) You should mainly feel the muscles working at the front of your thigh above your knee.

Quantity: Stretch each leg 6 times

Benefits: This exercise is as much a warm up as a stretch and helps work the thighs. While it mainly targets the quadriceps, it also helps stretch the inside of the thighs.

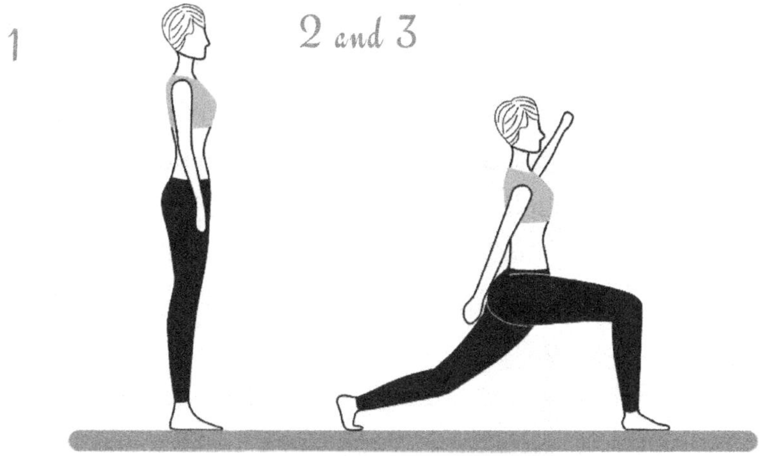
1
2 and 3

Stretch 24 - Legs-up-the-Wall Pose (Yoga)

This pose can be practiced by anyone, without any risk of injury.

1) Lie down on your back with your sit bones against the wall and your legs in the air against the wall. Your back should be resting on the ground without arching. Keep your body symmetrical and your pelvis parallel to the wall. Place your hands on your stomach. Feel your spine stretch.
2) Stretch your legs and try to point your toes toward you (this will lift your heels slightly off the wall). *Take 6 deep breaths*. Now point your feet. *Take 6 deep breaths. Do 3 sets.*
3) Open your legs out as wide as possible without hurting yourself. Keep your legs straight and point your toes toward you. *Take 6 deep breaths. On each exhale, try to open your legs wider.*
4) Return to position 2), then rotate your legs to bring your heels toward your pubis, placing the soles of your feet together. Your calves and thighs should stay in contact with the wall. *Do 6 breathing cycles.* Then return to position 2) before pulling away from the wall and straightening up.

If you have spent the day on your feet or it is particularly hot, you can repeat this sequence several times, or even hold a position for several minutes.

Benefits: If you suffer from swollen legs, then this is the exercise for you. *For maximum effect, don't hesitate to combine it with other tips and tricks to help drain and stimulate your lymphatic system (see the 2nd part of this book).*

2

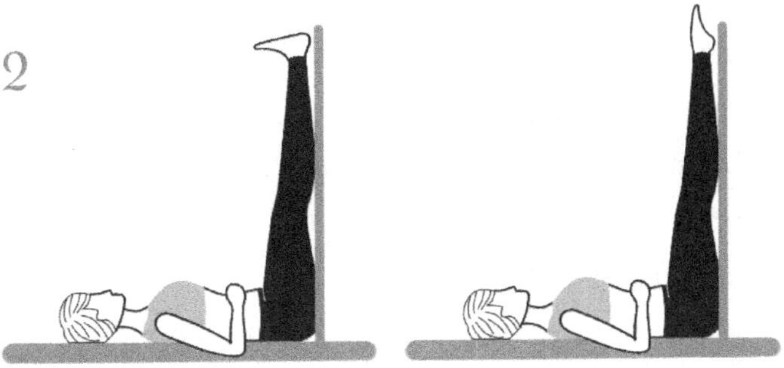

3 4

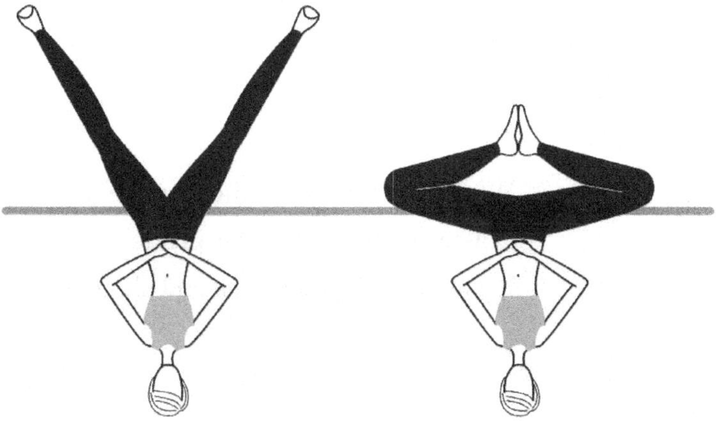

Stretch 25 - Revolved Side-Angle Pose (Yoga)

1) Start in Mountain pose. Keep your left leg still and slide your right leg backward, with your hands on your hips. Your left foot should point forward and your left leg should be bent, while your right foot points outward and your right leg is straight. Your left knee should be above your ankle (not your toes).
2) Lean your torso toward your left thigh, until it is aligned with your right leg. Lift your right arm up above your head, so it is also aligned with your torso, and turn your palm down toward the ground. Place your left hand on the ground, behind your foot. Your torso should be resting on your thigh. Try to move the left side of your butt back toward your right foot. Keep your left hand light: most of your body weight should be on your left leg. *Hold the pose for 6 deep breaths.*
3) Repeat on the other side.

Benefits: While this pose uses the muscles of the bent leg, it also helps stretch the inside of your extended leg as well as your sides and shoulders.

1

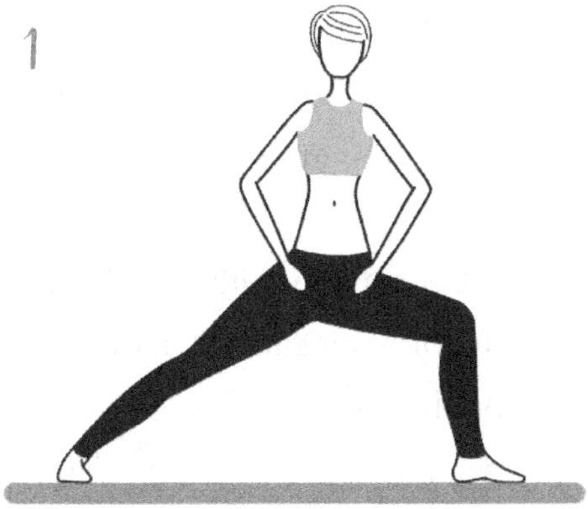

2

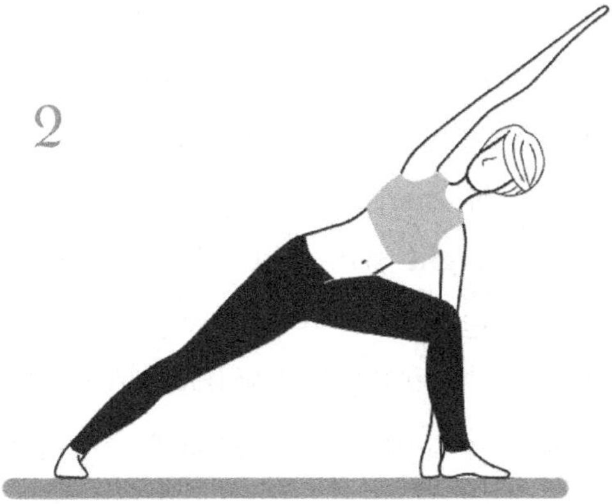

Stretch 26 - Revolved Half Moon Pose (Yoga)

1) Stand with your legs hip width apart and your knees soft.
2) Lean gently forward, hinging only at your hips, until your body is parallel to the ground and you can put your hands on the floor.
3) Keep your left hand in contact with the ground, and put your right hand on your sacrum, as you bend your right leg and gradually slide your left leg back. *Your body weight should now be resting on your right leg and left arm.*
4) As you straighten your right knee, keeping only the fingers of your left hand on the ground, slowly raise your left leg until it is in line with your back (parallel to the floor). Your toes should be pointing down to the ground. Open your chest and raise your right arm until it is aligned with your left arm. Lift your gaze up to your right hand. *If you find it hard to stay balanced, look down at your left hand.*
5) Lower your right arm and left leg down to the ground again, bending your knees slightly.
6) Lift your torso until you are back in the starting position. Repeat the exercise, raising your right leg and left arm.

Practicing this exercise barefoot will allow you to feel the ground better and keep your balance. Don't forget to breathe deeply throughout the exercise.

If you are worried about falling or if you need to improve your balance, I suggest you do this exercise against a wall: you can rest the hand that is raised toward the ceiling against the wall to help you balance.

Quantity: Hold the pose for 6 deep abdominal breaths on each side.

Benefits: This pose helps strengthen and tone the legs. Twisting the torso also works the abdominals. Given the current way of life in the West, it certainly has its interest...

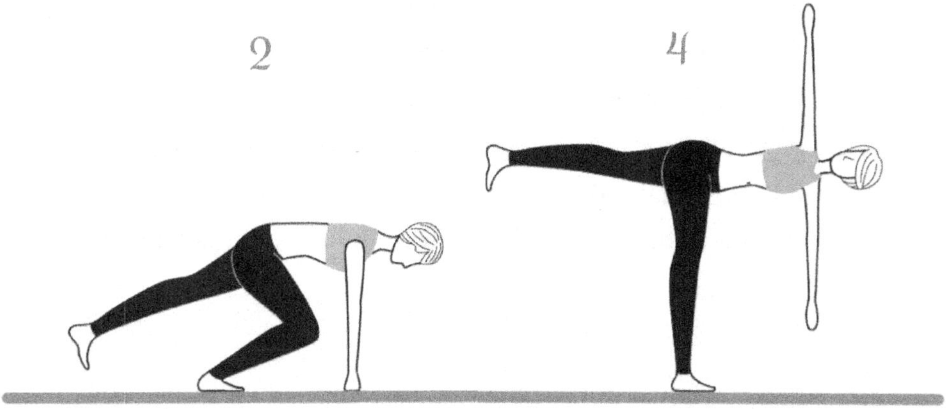

Stretch 27 - Intense Side Stretch (Yoga)

1) Starting in Mountain Pose, bring your shoulders forward to help you slide your hands up your back, palm to palm with the edge of your hands against your spine, until they are level with your heart. Your elbows should be pointing backward.
2) Now take a step back with your left foot. Your feet should be hip width apart, and your left foot pointing slightly outward for better stability. *Do 2 breathing cycles.*
3) On an exhale, bend forward from the hips, keeping your neck relaxed. Rest your forehead on your right tibia. Your legs should be firm and straight. *Do 6 breathing cycles.* With each inhale, try to lengthen your spine further, as though your head is being drawn toward the ground and your sit bones are being drawn up toward the ceiling.
4) On an exhale, raise yourself gently back up again. Bring your left foot back beside your right foot in Mountain Pose. Repeat on the other side.

Benefits: Ideal for stretching the hips and opening the shoulders. The forward bend stretches the back of the legs and massages the organs.

1

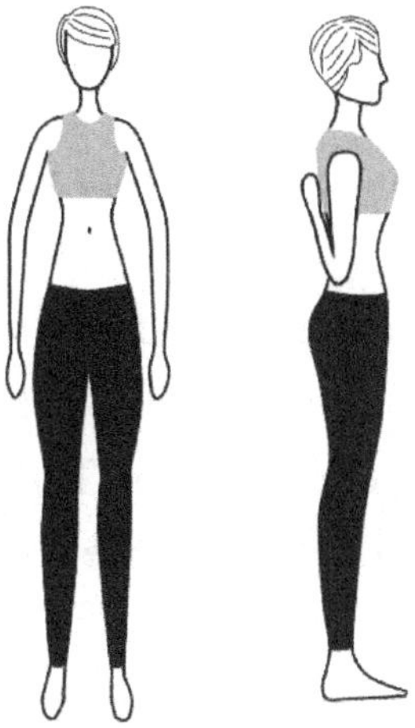

2

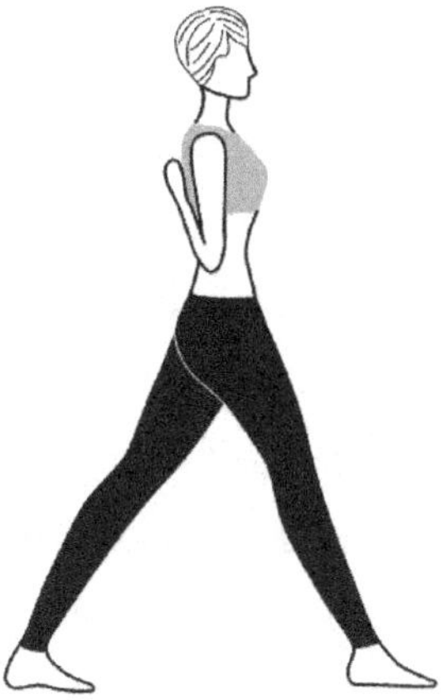

3

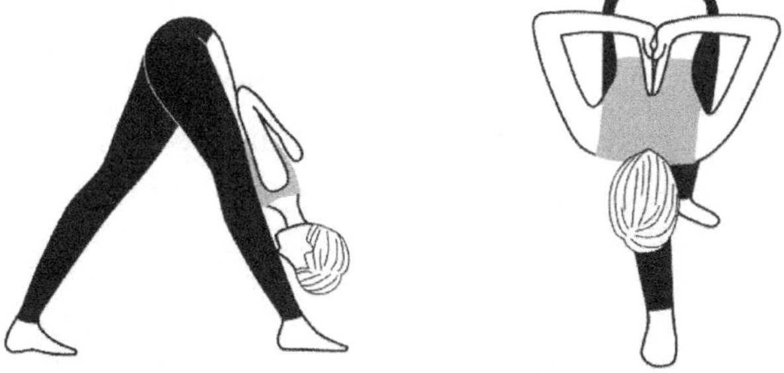

Stretch 28 - Seated Forward Fold with Toe Stretch (Yoga)

1) Begin sitting with your legs crossed, with your right leg in front of your left leg.
2) Lean slightly forward and intertwine the fingers of your right hand with the toes of your left foot, and the fingers of your left hand with the toes of your right foot. Tighten your hands to squeeze your toes slightly. Your heels should be down on the ground.
3) On an exhale, lean forward, extending your spine until your forehead is resting on the floor and your elbows by your sides. Make sure your butt does not lift from the floor. *Do 6 breathing cycles, centering within.*
4) On an inhale, sit gently back up again, release your feet, and change position, putting your left leg in front of your right leg. Repeat.

Benefits: After wearing tight shoes all day long, this exercise helps release any tension from the feet, especially the toes.

1

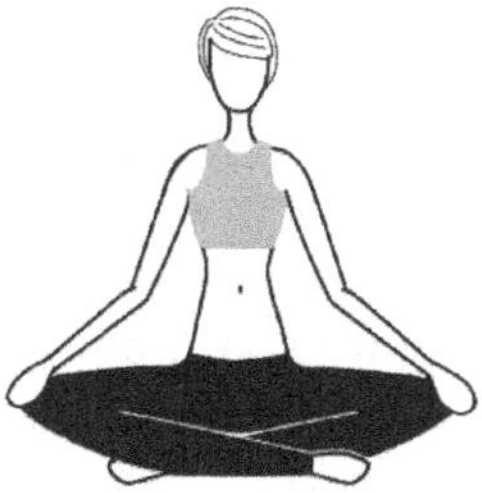

2

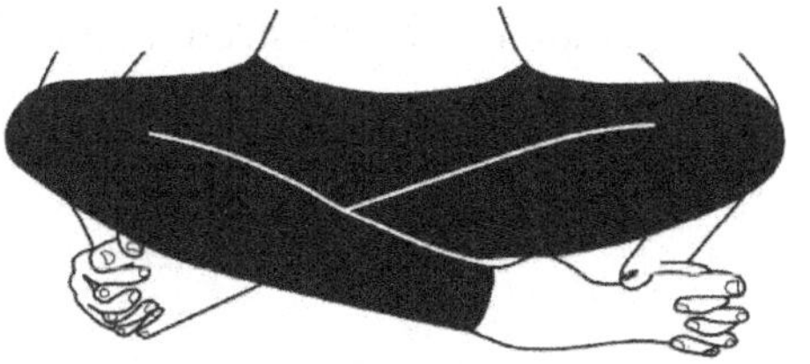

3

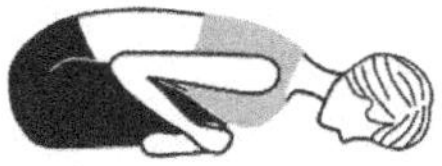

Stretch 29 - Toe Bend and Stretch

1) Sit down on the floor, supporting yourself with your hands. Keep your shoulders low, your chest broad, and your legs together.
2) Curl your toes as far as you can (this will push the soles of your feet toward you). *Hold for 6 seconds.*
3) Return to the starting position, then spread your toes as far apart as possible. *Hold for 6 seconds.*
4) Do 6 sets of step 2), and then 6 sets of step 3), holding for several seconds each time. Then do several quick sets.

Benefits: This sequence helps stretch and relax the toes and the soles of the feet.

1

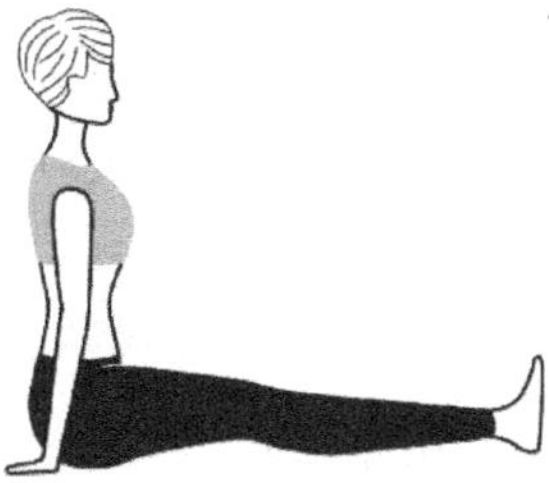

2

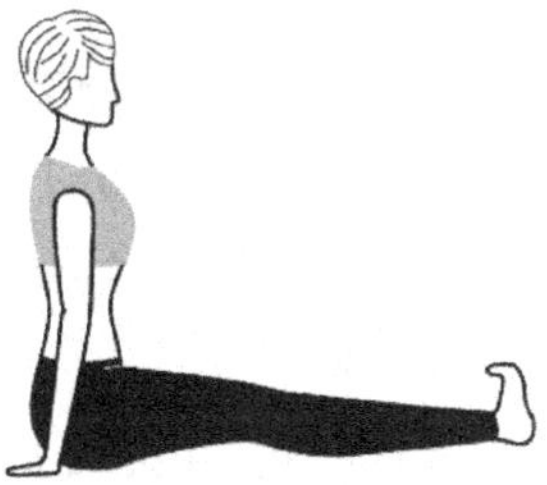

3

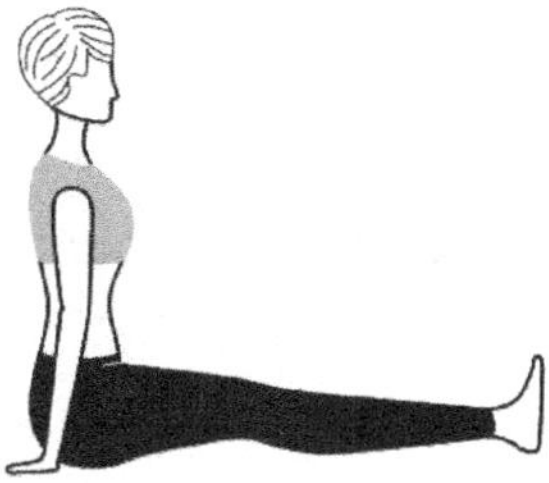

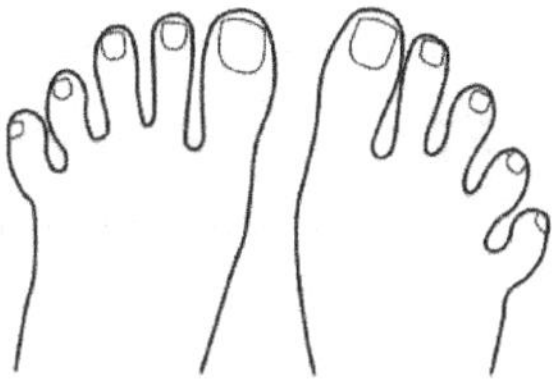

Stretch 30 - Foot Circles

1) Sit down on the floor, supporting yourself with your hands. Keep your shoulders low, your chest broad, and your legs together.
2) Draw circles with your feet (as wide as possible), keeping them both together, first in a clockwise direction and then in an anti-clockwise direction. *Do 6 rotations in each direction.*
3) Spread your legs hip width apart and work each foot separately, making circles in a clockwise direction and then in an anti-clockwise direction. *Do 6 rotations in each direction with each foot.*

Benefits: This exercise targets the ankles, helping to stretch and loosen them.

1

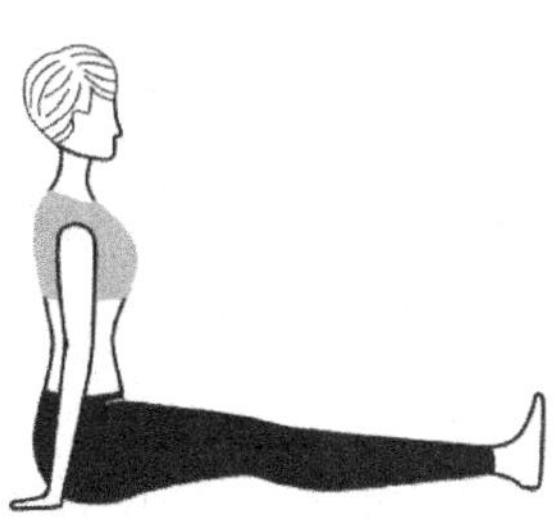

2

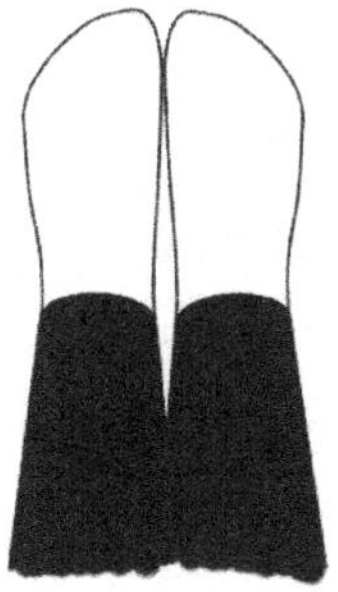

3

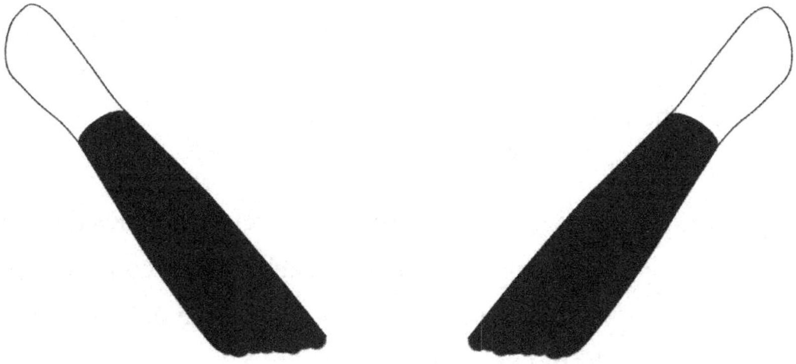

Stretch 31 - Heel to Butt

1) Kneel up on the floor with your legs hip width apart, your body aligned with your thighs and at right angles to your calves, and your hands on your hips. Only your knees and toes should be in contact with the ground.
2) On an exhale, lower your butt down as close as possible to your heels, keeping your back straight. Some people may even be able to sit on their heels.
3) On an inhale, engage your abdominals and glutes to return to the starting position. *Do 5 sets and then, if you can, stay sitting on your heels for 6 breathing cycles.*
4) Return to the starting position. Now place your feet flat against the ground. Repeat the same exercise as before. *Do 5 sets and then, if you can, stay sitting on your heels for 6 breathing cycles.*

Don't hesitate to put a small blanket under your knees if they get sore, and a yoga brick or dictionary between your feet to rest your butt on if the pose is difficult or painful.

Benefits: The first variant of this exercise stretches the toes and soles of the feet, and the second variant stretches the tops of the feet. The ankles benefit from this exercise too!

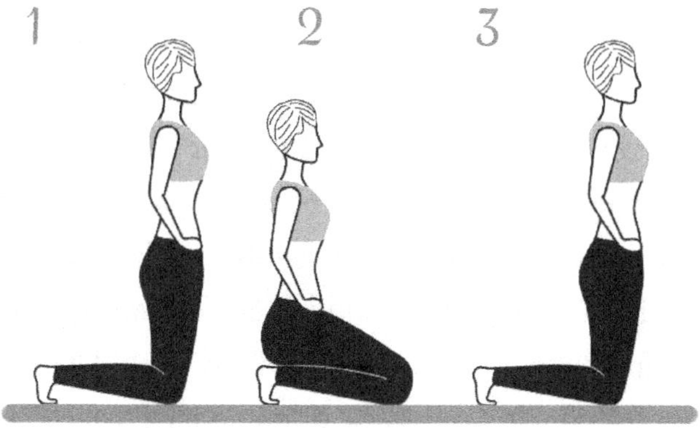
1
2
3

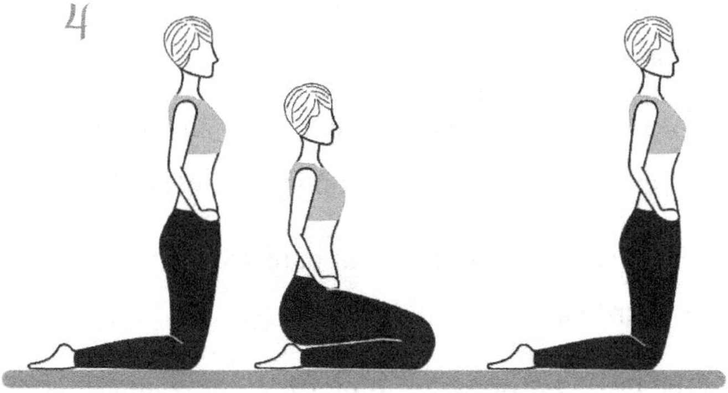
4

Stretch 32 – Tree Pose (Yoga)

1) Starting in Mountain pose, transfer your body weight onto your right leg, keeping it straight and firm.
2) Bend your left knee and rotate your leg to bring the sole of your left foot up against the inside of your right knee. At the same time, bring your hands together into a salutation, with your thumbs touching your sternum at your heart (the heart chakra). The top of your body should be relaxed, with no tension in your neck or shoulders, your chin straight, and your gaze distant or your eyes closed if you are more experienced. *Hold the pose for 6 breathing cycles (or more if you feel confident).*
3) Repeat the exercise transferring your body weight onto your left leg.

Variant for the legs: raise your bent leg so that the sole of your foot is against the inside of your thigh, and your heel against your groin.

Variant for the arms: Keeping your hands together, raise your arms up above your head.

To hold the pose, empty your mind of any unwanted thoughts.

Benefits: This is THE pose for working your balance, and to keep your balance you work your feet and ankles. You can also use this pose for meditation.

1

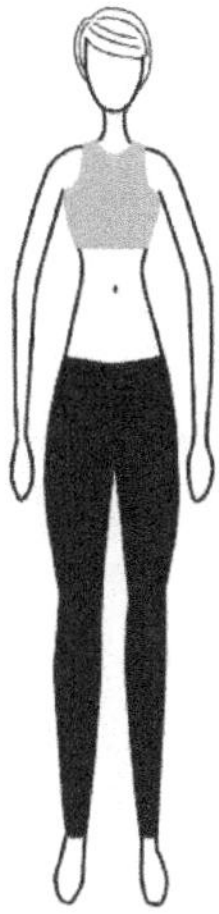

2

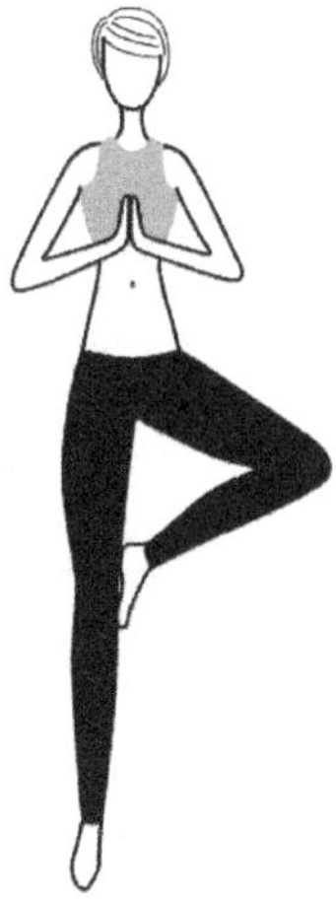

Variant

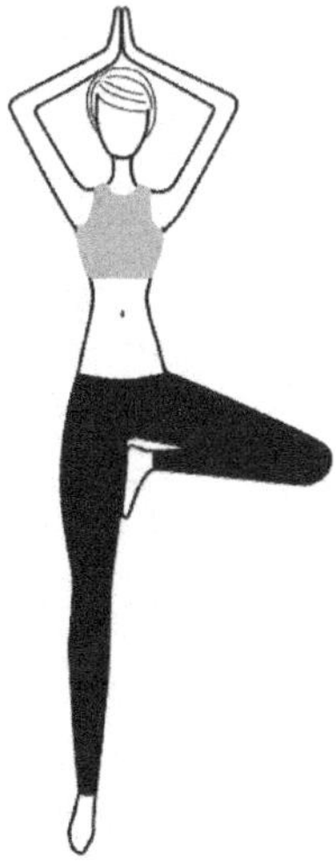

- Chapter 18 -
How to End the Session

After a few exercises (and a long day!), there is nothing like enjoying a few minutes to relax, unwind, and even meditate.

Here we will just look at one pose, the easiest pose of all.

Corpse Pose (Yoga)

> Lie down on the floor, with your neck clear, your arms a little distance from your body, and your legs slightly apart. Stay like this for a few minutes.

This pose is even more beneficial if you use conscious abdominal breathing (inflate your belly on the inhale, and deflate your belly on the exhale).

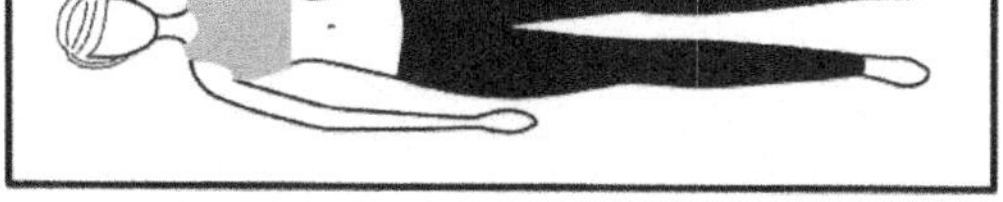

Summary Table of Exercises and Stretches

	PAGE	POSE	TO WORK THE...				
			Neck and shoulders	**Back and spine**	**Abdomen**	**Hips and Pelvis**	**Butt**
WARM UP	120	1 - The Back, Chest, and Shoulders					
	122	2 - The Spine					
	124	3 - The Neck					
	126	4 - The Neck					
	128	5 - The Hips					
EXERCISES	132	1 - The Stairs					
	134	2 - Pliés/Relevés					
	136	3 - The Dragonfly					
	138	4 - Strengthening the		Lumbar spine	Abdominals		
		Abdominals and Lower Back					
STRETCHES	144	1 - Opposite Arm and Leg Extension					
	146	2 - Sun Salutation (Y)					
	148	3 - Cat Pose					
	150	4 - Knee to Chest		Lumbar spine			
	152	5 - Ankle to Hand		Lumbar spine	Sides		
	154	6 - Revolved Abdomen Pose (Y)		Lumbar spine			
	156	7 - The Lying Half Lotus		Lumbar spine			
	158	8 - The Butterfly					
	160	9 - Cobbler's Pose (Y)					
	162	10 - Standing Forward Bend (Y)		Lumbar spine			
	164	11 - Grand Plié in Second				Hips	
	166	12 - The Frog					
	168	13 - Cross-Legged Forward Fold (Y)					
	170	14 - Crescent Moon Pose (Y)					
	172	15 - Chest to Thigh				Hips	
	174	*Variant* 16 - Chest over Crossed Thighs				Hips	
	176	17 - Downward Dog (Y)					
	178	18 - Extended Hand-to-Big-Toe Pose (Y)					

TO WORK THE...						
Legs	**Knees**	**Ankles**	**Feet**	**Balance**	**Blood circulation**	**And also...**
Calves						
Thighs						
						Concentration
						Massages the organs
Inner thighs						Circulation of energy in the pelvis
Back of legs and thighs					Head	Concentration
Thighs						
Inner thighs						Meditation
Front of the thighs						Revitalizes the liver and kidneys
Back of the legs						
Inner thighs and calves						
Back of the thighs					Head	

	PAGE	POSE	TO WORK THE...				
			Neck and shoulders	**Back and spine**	**Abdomen**	**Hips and Pelvis**	**Butt**
STRETCHES	180	19 - The Perfect Pose (Y)					
	182	20 - Single-Leg-Folded Seated Forward Fold (Y)					
	184	21 - Head-to-Knee with Stretched Toes Pose (Y)					
	186	22 - Inverted Splits					
	188	23 - Lunge					
	190	24 - Legs-up-the-Wall Pose (Y)					
	192	25 - Revolved Side-Angle Pose (Y)			Sides		
	194	26 - Revolved Half Moon Pose (Y)			Abdominals		
	196	27 - Intense Side Stretch (Y)					
	198	28 - Seated Forward Fold with Toe Stretch					
	200	29 - Toe Bend and Stretch					
	202	30 - Foot Circles					
	204	31 - Heel to Butt					
	206	32 - Tree Pose (Y)					

TO WORK THE...						
Legs	**Knees**	**Ankles**	**Feet**	**Balance**	**Blood circulation**	**And also...**
					Lumbar spine and genitals	
						Revitalizes the organs, Sciatica
Back of the thighs		Achilles tendons				Revitalizes the organs
Back of the legs						
Thighs						
Back of the legs					Legs	
						Revitalizes the abdomen
Back of the legs						Revitalizes the organs
			Toes			Revitalizes the organs

Appendix

The Emergency Kit to Keep in any Handbag

Here is a non-exhaustive list of products to keep in your handbag. Sooner or later you'll find they come in handy for all sorts of purposes, not just your feet.

1 spare pair of ballerina shoes - If your feet are tired and bruised, or if you need to walk fast because you are in a hurry. Try the Rollasole or Bagllerina brands for a pair of foldable shoes.

1 plastic bag – So you can store your shoes (spare ballerina shoes or painful pumps) in your bag without making them dirty.

2 antiseptic dressings – Cuts and grazes can happen easily, and carrying an antiseptic spray that can leak in your bag isn't a great idea. Of course, this is just until you get home to disinfect the wound properly.

2 hydrocolloid dressings - Useful in the case of blisters.

Some tampons or sanitary towels

1 tube of Arnica 9c homeopathy - Essential if you tend to bump yourself (to make sure your shins aren't covered in bruises) or if your muscles are aching. Take 5 granules (to be renewed 3 to 5 times a day).

1 tube of Oscillococcinum – Is it flu season? Are you aching and feverish? Quick, take a tube!

Mint drops, dental floss, and maybe even a travel toothbrush and toothpaste - Choose according to how much space you have left in your kit or bag.

1 small deodorant

1 perfume sample - In case you forgot to put perfume on in the morning or it has worn off by the end of the day.

1 lip balm or lip oil and lipstick

1 nail file

1 spare pair of tights or stockings

List of Precautions for Use and Contraindications

Remember that the cosmetic recipes and formulas described in this book, as well as the products they are made of, are only intended for external use on the skin by an adult (with the exception of women who are pregnant or breastfeeding, who must not use or touch them, as with children). Moreover, they must be kept out of the reach of children.

The recipes described in this book and the products they are made of should not be applied on or near the eyes or mucous membranes, nor ingested or inhaled/diffused.

The list of precautions for use and contraindications that follows is not exhaustive and only concerns the external use of the products described on the skin. If you have any doubts or questions, consult your doctor or pharmacist.

None of the recipes described in this book, or their constituents, are to be used over an extended period without medical advice.

In general, always do a skin test for each product or recipe by placing a few drops over a 1 inch area in the crook of your elbow 48 hours before using it. If you feel any itching or notice the slightest redness or any other reaction (tingling, difficulty breathing, etc.), do not use it.

When you have finished making a recipe, always do a pH test. If needed, you can adjust the recipe with baking soda.

Recipe 1:

Baking soda:

- Do not store baking soda mixed with acidic products in a closed container.

Citric acid:

- Do not forget to put on protective gloves and goggles before handling.

Kpangnan butter:

- Be careful not to burn yourself when handling the melted wax.

Bay leaf vegetable oil:

- Intended for external use only, it should not be used pure on the skin but diluted in a neutral vegetable oil or in a recipe.
- This vegetable oil contains essential oils.
- Do not use this oil in the case of allergies to bay or asteraceae (chamomile, calendula, etc.) because of the presence of sesquiterpene lactones.

Lemongrass essential oil:

- The citral (geranium and neral), citronellol, geraniol, iso-eugenol, limonene, and linalool in this essential oil can cause allergies in some sensitive people.

- This essential oil is considered dermocaustic and an irritatant to the skin and can cause an allergic reaction in external use, especially if not diluted.

Pink peppercorn essential oil:

- The limonene in this essential oil can cause allergies in some sensitive people.
- Do not use pure on the skin: it should always be diluted in a vegetable oil.
- This warming essential oil can be an irritant.
- Avoid using this essential oil on the face.
- Avoid contact with the eyes.

Recipe 2:

Clary sage essential oil:

- Not recommended if you have a history of endocrine disorders (such as excess estrogen), mastosis, or hormone-dependent cancer, either personally or in your family. Ask your doctor for advice.
- The limonene and linalool in this essential oil can cause allergies in some sensitive people.

Mediterranean Cyprus essential oil:

- The limonene and linalool in this essential oil can cause allergies in some sensitive people.

- Not recommended if you have a history of hormone-dependent cancer, either personally or in your family. Ask your doctor for advice.

Rose geranium essential oil:

- The citral (neral and geranium), citronellol, geraniol, limonene, and linalool in this essential oil can cause allergies in some sensitive people.

Recipe 3:

Aloe vera gel:

- Unless otherwise stated under the sole liability of the manufacturer, Aloe Vera gel is a cosmetic product, not suitable for food use.

Butcher's broom extract:

- Respect the recommended doses.

Peppermint essential oil:

- This essential oil is considered an irritant and coolant when applied to the skin, and can cause an allergic reaction through external use, especially if not diluted (the maximum concentration of peppermint essential oil in a composition should not exceed 30%).
- Not to be used by epileptics or the elderly.

- The limonene, linalool, and menthol in this essential oil can cause allergies in some sensitive people.
- This essential oil is neurotoxic and narcotic in high doses, and can also cause insomnia, ataxia, tremors, bradycardia and headaches.

Mastic essential oil:

- This essential oil is considered dermocaustic and an irritant to the skin and can cause an allergic reaction through external use, especially if it is not diluted.
- The limonene and linalool in this essential oil can cause allergies in some sensitive people.

Grapefruit seed extract:

- Respect the recommended doses.
- Do not apply pure to the skin.

Recipe 4:

Kokum butter:

- Be careful not to burn yourself when handling the melted butter.

Shea butter:

- Shea butter naturally contains latex and is to be avoided in the case of a latex allergy.
- Be careful not to burn yourself when handling the melted butter.

Jasmin Grandiflorum wax:

- The benzyl alcohol, benzyl benzoate, linalool, and benzyl salicylate in this essential oil can cause allergies in some sensitive people.
- Be careful not to burn yourself when handling the melted wax.

Ylang-Ylang essential oil:

- Avoid applying this essential oil pure to the skin, as it is considered a dermocaustic skin irritant, especially in the case of sensitive skin.
- The benzyl benzoate, citral, eugenol, farnesol, geraniol, linalool, and benzyl salicylate in this essential oil can cause allergies in some sensitive people.

Neroli essential oil:

- The farnesol, geraniol, limonene, and linalool in this essential oil can cause allergies in some sensitive people.

Recipe 5:

Katafray essential oil:

- Avoid if you suffer from allergies and/or have sensitive skin.
- The limonene in this essential oil can cause allergies in some sensitive people.

Lavandin Super essential oil:

- Not advised if you are epileptic.
- The limonene and linalool in this essential oil can cause allergies in some sensitive people.

Recipe 6:

Sweet almond milk powder:

- Not recommended if you are allergic to nuts.
- A powder product, keep away from sources of ventilation, and do not inhale. Wear protective goggles, gloves, apron, and dust mask when handling.

Damask rose powder:

- A powder product, keep away from sources of ventilation, and do not inhale. Wear protective goggles, gloves, apron, and dust mask when handling.
- According to Ayurveda, it can increase "inner fire" in high doses.

Honey powder:

- A powder product, keep away from sources of ventilation, and do not inhale. Wear protective goggles, gloves, apron, and dust mask when handling.

Allantoin powder:

- A powder product, keep away from sources of ventilation, and do not inhale. Wear protective goggles, gloves, apron, and dust mask when handling.
- Respect the recommended doses.

Centella asiatica powder:

- A powder product, keep away from sources of ventilation, and do not inhale. Wear protective goggles, gloves, apron, and dust mask when handling.

Notes

First legal registration (French version): November 2016

Legal registration (English version): September 2017

Printed by: CreateSpace, USA

Made in United States
Orlando, FL
16 February 2024

43774108R00134